Full Circle

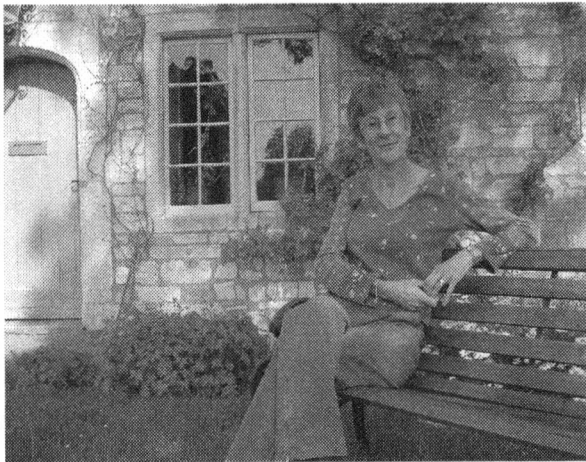

By Pauline Pearce

Published by:
Chipmunka publishing
PO Box 6872
Brentwood
Essex
CM13 1ZT
United Kingdom

www.chipmunkapublishing.com

ISBN 978 1 84747 014 0

The development of this book was made possible by a grant from The Arts Council, London.

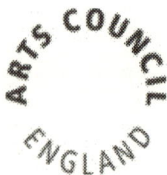

PREFACE:

This is my story written from the heart.

It might, initially, be an uncomfortable read but this is my unabridged story- the truth of my life as it was as an adolescent and into early adulthood.

Some might say, perhaps, it would have been better unwritten - that, in many ways, I am exposing something too personal that should remain within me rather than in written, exposing words. Yet, I feel no shame in the text I have penned.

My greatest desire, is to give something to others in emotional or physical distress - that out despair can come hope; that out of weakness can come strength.

This is the message of my book. I hope that I have achieved this in the words I have written.

This would not have been penned without the support given to me by my family - my husband; my beautiful daughter (of whom I am so proud); a girl's best friend (my mum) and, last but not least, my sister and her husband. I thank each one of you and dedicate this book to you, with the greatest of love.

Part 1: DESPERATELY SEEKING "PAULINE"

Chapter 1.

Why do I feel so sad?

I have so much to be thankful for – a loving husband; a beautiful, teenage daughter; a comfortable home, in a rural Cheshire village, and - as a bonus - am sitting in the hot sunshine on a veranda overlooking the Amalfi coast, one of the most scenic views in, not only Italy but in the entire world. Then, why sad? Why are tears just a nano-second away?

Why if I could just doze off in the heat, in the beauty of the surroundings never to re-awaken, why might that feel so good?

I'm tired – not tired of life in general – that has potential, new experience, new adventure ahead. No, I'm tired of my life and the constant fight I feel everyday is becoming. I'm 45, yet sometimes I feel doubly this, as I strive not wanting to give in to the illness and pain, both physical & psychologically, that constantly exhausts me. Now would be a good time for an ending – in the warm sunshine, in these beautiful surroundings before life becomes more burdensome and my capabilities become more limited. Before my life shrinks any more.

I've never quite understood why so often, on war memorials, mention is made to the sadness of young men cut off in their prime, yet - as a positive – their bodies never ageing. They'll be remembered at the age they met their maker – for the beauty of their youth; for the life potential they had, yet didn't fulfill; for the perfection of their fit, young bodies.

I'm scared of death (even though a Christian) – the uncertainties, the finality but, perhaps more, the mode and shape of its advent. I've seen too many friends near my own age die recently. I've watched their gradual deterioration, their loss of dignity as illness stripped them of mobility and independence – bed pans, bed baths, loss of control of bowels and bladder; returning both in body and mind to infancy. That scares me.

Yet, what of my future? Do I want to cling on to life by the tips of my fingernails, knowing I may endure this? Is this deterioration happening, as I pen this paper? I feel so. Life is different now. Little by little, quality is ebbing away, no matter how hard I try to maintain normality as it once was.

I'm living a fool's paradise. I push myself, often beyond my limits, trying to prove this quality is still there. It's the uncertainty of my illness and, maybe it's progression that scares me. How far will it deteriorate? How bad will it get? Why is it so unpredictable and no one can give me any definite answers? I push myself for my family – for my husband and daughter, even for myself. I want them to see me (and me to feel) as normal as possible and that we, as a family, don't have to change our established routine – evolved over the past 16 years. But it's not really working. I see this but do they also?

Sometimes, despite my fear of death and possible nothingness - this illness has even challenged my faith of life eternal. Sometimes, I feel I'd just like to slip away but it would have to be gentle; kind to me; unknowingly planned, like slipping into sleep with, (as now,) the Ravello church bells chiming, in the gentle sunshine and quiet breeze. Not for me, the planned self-euthanasia of pills or toxic fumes. Those days are long gone. That was the old selfish me. Yet how can I slip away even if I prayed hard enough for this? What about those left behind – husband, child? I know, at times, they are intolerant and frustrated at my limitations and show it, which hurts so much. They suffer too because of my illness. I can't do what I was once able to for my daughter – ferrying her to friends houses; shopping trips; swimming together - all precious times of bonding, of getting to know one another better. Yes, mum's still "around" but I feel like a shell - *a vacuum. The body and* mind's still there but so much of the physical capabilities gone. Part of me - and often the part my daughter wants most, has gone. Maybe never to return.

I sound like a spoilt child now, but I **want,** I **need** that "filling" back – energy, physical capability. She's only here now (pre-university) for 2 more years. I want to give her more of me; the physicality; this part of me during these years. Yet, I feel it going. It's ebbing away and I've no control.

Husband needs far more from me than I feel daughter does. Physical presence I can give but again the shell's there – the vacuum overwhelms the body. I get so tired of the constant fight with muscles with a will of their own; the embarrassment I try to hide; the pills that scramble my brains. They affect my balance, my eye-sight, my memory, my fluency of speech. I don't feel like a whole person any more. I don't feel like a person with much to give my family – only to cause worry and concern to those I love most.

But, what for me is the answer to this? Become fatalistic? "Que cera, cera?" Wait for further infirmity to develop on an unknown time scale? Sit back, eliminating progress of infirmity from mind. Pray for a miracle cure that will return me to normality?

That is not me, or rather, not me now. That was the "old me" of previous years. Infirmity gave me a reason not to succeed. Infirmity was an escape from normal life and adult psychological growth. Infirmity, especially that of the mind, meant no-one expected anything from me – academic achievement; self-responsibility; ability to cope with my own flesh and blood infant. Infirmity made me special. It even made me, in the most ironic of ways, important. I didn't need academic degrees or a responsible job. I was the centre of attention without any of these – the more I self-harmed; the more intoxicated I became – the more attention I got and craved. I learnt these lessons from an early age, when hospitalised at 16 years old, under the diagnostic term of nervous breakdown, observing and then replicating behaviour of my new circle of companions. The schizophrenics; the psychotics; the old women who'd been admitted to mental asylums in their teens, merely for the crime of giving birth to bastard children. Yes, perhaps in the true sense of madness, these women were now insane. But, originally in their tender years of late childhood, the only crime they'd been persecuted and locked away for, was for pre-marital pregnancy when the gin bottle or other barbaric forms of self-mutilation or back-street abortion had failed.

That place - that asylum (thank God, they don't exist any more in this country) became my home, even my sanctuary, for several years. It separated me, with its prison like walls and inward stench of urine, from that fearful - as it became to me - world beyond. I feared the asylum and its inmates but I feared the real world much more.

I developed ways of coping that made the asylum, less fearful for me. The bad girls – the self-harmers with razor or broken glass slashed arms

– slept near the nurses' office, on the ground floor. If you were deemed in better psychological health, you were shunted up to the dormitories with the mad old women, where the nurses ventured less often. Here, the stench of urine and faeces was overpowering. The windows were tight closed and locked, for fear an elderly chrone, drugged and disorientated, might try to fly to freedom. I use the word old-chrone or hag which terminology now abhors me, but that is how at 16, I viewed these old women. If not drugged up sufficiently (tolerance to medication over the years, having built up) these hags would wander up and down the dormitories, chanting and raving undistinguishingly, hour upon hour. Sometimes, in disorientation, they'd climb into an already occupied bed. Fights between chrones often ensued, until nurses, usually male, pulled them apart and forcibly injected some soporific medication.

I prayed daily, to some or other deity – how could there possibly be a God? - not, to be thought of as better. Cutting arms; hoarding medication; getting drunk on illicit alcohol was, for me, far better than nights of purgatory and intense fear, upstairs, where few nurses ventured.

Yet one day, I went too far. Did I kick a nurse? I was put in a padded cell and stripped to my underwear. By now, I think embarrassment had been well and truly lost, in the blur of heavy medication. I remember a bed, a toilet, a small slit for a window, which gave little light. I was allowed no visitors. Would I want any? Time meant nothing to me. I must have been fed and watered and I do remember painful injections being administered. I think I slept for most of this time. I know my parents were unhappy with my treatment but they, over-awed by the consultant psychiatrist and his advice, perhaps thought he knew what was best for me, at this time. They so wanted their daughter returned to them sane and back to some sort of normality.

I think I was in this cell for 7 days or so. The psychiatrist thought I'd taken my punishment well. I perceive he increased or altered my medication and sent me to see the psychologist who, in my memory, was the first kind individual there I can remember, and was instrumental in my discharge from this hell-hole.

I want, now, to look at the "crime" that took me to this barbaric institution. Otherwise, even at this point in my life, having closed these doors for many years, and now in re-opening them briefly, I wonder, was I insane? .

Chapter 2

The story began when I was 15 years old. I was a solitary child , my sister being 10 years older did not always want the companionship of an annoying, younger sibling. In retrospect, quite understandable from her perspective but not, at that time, as a little sister. She married when I was 12 years old and soon left the roots of her home city. For most of her adult life, the mode of her husband's employment made them almost "nomadic" as each promotion took them from one area of the UK another.

We - mother, father, self - lived in a large, quite isolated house in an affluent suburb of Liverpool. I had no friends of my own age living nearby and school friends were not often encouraged to visit. My mother had a philosophy – home was meant to sparkle, to shine; to be kept in tidy perfection. Young children and later, teenagers, made mess. They took the shine off immaculately polished wood block floors. They trampled the pile on expensive Chinese carpets. Mother spent all day with Betty the daily help, polishing, sweeping, washing down already pristine paint work, and plumping up sofa cushions that anyone might dare to have sat on.
I admit to behaving similarly, in early days of marriage - forever the perfectionist - much to my shame now! "Like mother, like daughter"!

From, it seems like infancy, I – with nothing better to do - followed what I thought was a normal pattern. After polishing surfaces to perfection, I, when small in stature, would stand on a kitchen stool, washing and scrubbing underpants and socks that mother denied could be properly cleaned in the washing machine.

I don't remember a lot of my father up until about the age of 12. I remember being slightly afraid of his temper and the consequences of not finishing a meal. This came from the poverty of his background and of all food being extremely precious and not to be wasted. I also remember, my mother being in hospital for 3 weeks, following an operation, and of being alone in the house (my sister now married) with what, at the time, felt a little like a stranger.

I think the stranger scenario, came from the fact that he, in all probability, was a workaholic but, in the sense of wanting to provide the best for his family. My father was financially very generous and, lucky child, he even bought me a pony at one point in my younger years. Every little girl's dream. From humble beginnings, he had studied long years in his youth to, eventually, become an accountant and a man of "standing". One of his favoured locations was the Golf Club and afterwards the "19th hole". He would often come home (pre-breathalyser days?) from this location for his Sunday lunch, in a most jovial mood. In this routine, then followed his Sunday afternoon rest. He was a man most happy in a schedule of set pattern of weekly routine.

I suppose, initially, because I was isolated in my home location and also, perhaps, craved a little more attention from my busy parents, when I first began school at the age of 5, it became my haven. It was a small private school. I had friends of my own age; teachers who genuinely seemed to care for their charges and, the biggest bonus for me, at this time, I shone academically. I had now become "special" and my parents were made aware of this too. They began to notice me, a little more and I liked it.

Yet, fate then stepped in, in what, initially, seemed a fortuitous way but later may also have proved my downfall.   The headmistress, when I was 11 years old, suggested to my parents that my academic prowess could be better nurtured and matured, at a school of greater academic standing.

Five very unhappy years ensued. I became one of many academically bright children - many far more intelligent than myself. I was special no longer, though fought long and hard to remain so. This school made much of academic achievement but unless you were possibly, Oxford or Cambridge bound, the child within was not really valued. Little value was placed on effort or to the child's development as a whole person. Academic perfection, or "as near as damn it", was to be strived and looked for, in each child, to (in my scenario) the expense of all else.

I strived to the utmost and to the detriment of myself as this whole person - which I now know is all important. My whole life became a continual fight for academic success. There became little else - school, homework, exams. Yet, it was never enough and this message was not just self-fed but externally fed, by this institution.

At some point in time in 1971, illness crept upon me and, at first, neither I nor my parents, saw it developing. The conclusion, after many months of disregarding strange symptoms, I developed quite severe voice, head and neck tremors and, accompanying this, acute physical pain.

The diagnosis from the family GP was that I was experiencing a nervous breakdown and these symptoms progressed, the closer I came to sitting my GCE examinations. The medical answer was to medicate - valium, artane, mogadon - to get me to the point of taking these, as it was regarded, all-important examinations, on which my future depended.

I took those exams and surprisingly passed, though, perhaps not with the expected grades that would bring credit to the school. I took them drugged, disorientated but I passed and was not a total academic failure.

After my final exam, I locked myself away at home - made myself a prisoner in my own bedroom. It was safe. I felt I looked like a freak. Now the important criteria - the exams - had come and gone, I didn't have to face the taunts I had received at school because I looked strange - my head and neck contorted grotesquely. My friends sniggered when I read aloud in class. I had asked the teachers to excuse me from this, as my voice shook and vibrated, and my words became slurred but my appeal fell on deaf ears. I hated these embittered, old spinsters (as I saw them then) with vehemence to the extreme. Where was their compassion? Where was their care for me in this situation?

On leaving school, my neck contortions and tremor, deteriorating – my fear of being seen in the outside world progressively increased. My GP insisted the "heavy gang" be brought in. By this, I mean the psychiatrists. Again, my parents, out of genuine concern for me, co-operated with those who they perceived knew what was in my best interests.

Initially, physical tests were carried out with no cause or reason being found. Antiquated psychiatrists, heads bent solemnly together, pronounced my fate. These symptoms were ones of the mind, and of the worst kind, hospitalization would be the answer.

I remember being drugged into unconsciousness, as my fear at leaving the sanctuary of home was so great. I awoke in a psychiatric ward, in an old and crumbling general hospital. The possible treatments for my condition were then activated, one after another. Drugs, different drugs and then, more zombyfying drugs – to no avail These were the days when talking therapy, as we recognize it now, was not in vogue.

Sodium Pentathlon (the "truth drug") was then administered to loosen my tongue. They had a sense I was holding back on some dark and unsavoury secret, which was at the root of all this but none came forth. E.C.T. was administered - horrifying and scaring. I can still hear the noise of the E.C.T. trolley, clanking and jangling, as it came a little closer to my curtained-off bed. That noise is embedded in my brain and is one I wish I could relinquish. Still no results, from my numerous E.C.T treatments, other than leading to my further disorientation and feelings of unreality from "life outside" – whatever that was. I was now in the land of the "zombies" – feeling I had no control over my life and not really caring.

On this ward, after several weeks, I had the option of weekend leave, which I often chose to pass on. In this mental fuzz I felt safer being institutionalized than participating in life beyond the walls of my sanctuary.

There were fewer patients around at this time and less staff and often, the male and female wards amalgamated for daytime activities. There was, I thought, a lovely married couple, both nurses, who worked at the weekend. I looked on them, in the kindness they showed, as a substitute mum and dad. However, Mr Evans - I can still remember his name, his face, his poignant smell -dispelled my fantasy of a father figure. I remember his nauseous breath as he closed in "for the kill" as he, assaulted me in the quietness of a Sunday afternoon, tucked away in a cupboard where no one could see. I should have fought. I should have cried out. I hated it. I didn't tell anyone about this until quite recently because, I had somehow felt a misplaced guilt for it happening. Certainly, at the time of it taking place, I thought no-one would believe me and would, perhaps, think it associated with MY state of mind - a symptom of my, as they saw it,   attention seeking. I'm, now, certain that that was why this detestable man,   thought he would escape retribution.

Perhaps, at this point in my story, I should explain the true picture - only recently discovered - of what rocked and changed my life at the age of 16. It brought me from a position of being a reasonably intelligent teenager, with the potential for future success,both in relationships and in whatever career I might have chosen, to this hell on earth.

Chapter 3.

The crime for which I was incarcerated was for acquiring a then (in the early 70's) unrecognised neurological condition called Dystonia – a movement disorder similar to Parkinson or M.S. It is possibly genetically linked and affects an area of the brain called the basal ganglia. This misfires and sends out incorrect messages to muscles in the body inducing unbidden movement and tremor. It can be focal and affect only one part of the body. In my scenario, it has been the area around my neck, vocal chords and head or it can affect the body as a whole. The sufferer is contorted into many grotesque and painful positions. The brain, the intellect, the sufferer's capabilities remain intact but the outward appearance of (a cruel word used by many in my youth) a spastic, is a symptom, over which the individual has no control.

Leading neurologists have, in the last decade, recognized it as a physical disability. In years before a presentation of such inexplicable symptoms, was regarded by physicians, as a psychosomatic disorder. Hence, the patient was extricated from the realms of medical diagnosis into the vacuity of psychiatry. It was deemed as "all in the mind".

Sufferers cannot perish from Dystonia – not in a physical sense but some, having been convinced by psychiatrists that they , have the power to bring cessation to these symptoms, have suffered a cruel and torturous psychological "death". Many sufferers, having received such messages, have indeed proceeded to commit suicide – rather than live, stigmatised and shamed by physicians and family.

I felt this shame. I felt the contempt of those who attended me. I was 16, I was a child – a frightened lonely child in a world of adult condemnation. These physicians were the experts. What did I know? I didn't want attention – not attention of this kind. I wanted unconditional love and reassurance. I wanted to be like my peers - to take my "A" levels, to go to university. That had been my life-plan. Yet, this assumed need for attention was the diagnostic conclusion from the medical fraternity. Yet, why couldn't I bring cessation to these physical symptoms that made me feel so different, so grotesque? I wanted to blend into life - into life as I had known it in my early teens. I asked myself this question, over and again, but came to no conclusion.

I think when I felt most ashamed, most humiliated, was when I was on the receiving end of the dreaded ward round. I had to present myself at this, in person. I can remember my heart beating wildly within my chest, in fear, as my "turn" grew nearer. I'd knock and enter a soulless clinical room and immediately, all eyes were on me. It felt like a judge and jury court appearance with me as defendant on charge.

The psychiatrist, ancient yet revered by his juniors, sat in judgement dressed in long white coat and half-moon spectacles. They -my jury - sat around in a circle. They only spoke if bidden by the "judge". I sat on a hard wooden backed chair in the centre of the room. The discomfort of the chair and the fear of my condemners - psychologist, ward sister, occupational therapists, students increased my physical symptoms. My head would tremor; my spasms increase; my voice shake and falter, but this was seen as evidence, to my jurors, that my symptoms were psychosomatic and attention seeking. Why, when the occupational therapist was invited to give "evidence", why when I was more relaxed and less aware of being observed weaving those endless baskets or wicker stools, which filled the tedious days of "captivity", why were my symptoms less pronounced?

Didn't this prove, as the judge passed sentence, that my symptoms were self-induced ? I was guilty as charged. My sentence - to be committed to the ancient mental institution where the "no-hopers" had been sent for the past century – away from the city and general humanity , castigated to what seemed like some far-flung corner of civilisation. An assumption that I was a failure to be kept out of sight as an entity, under the management of this revered man – an admission of his own defeat. "Hide this shameful creature away. We can do no more and failure is best hidden away and removed from view."

That's how it felt to me, at this time. That's how my parents received it also and it broke their hearts. No longer was I a child to be proud of as their off-spring. Now, I was something quite different - bringing shame to self and family and needing to be hidden away. This was the message both they and I received, from those who knew better than we did - the professionals.

Hence, my months at this institution. Many people had never heard of "Rainhill". Even fewer had seen it or knew what went on behind those high red-brick walls. I felt, on my sentencing - shame; failure; worthless; thrown on the scrap-heap of life; maybe even subhuman.

Yet through one man – a psychologist - the person who gave me reprieve, after my time in "solitary", I made my escape from the "mad house".   However, after many years, of institutionalisation, the world beyond felt terrifying to the extreme. I felt safer in confinement, as brutal as it was, than in the world beyond.

I was sent to a half way house in a less than salubrious part of Manchester. Still drugs – drugs to sleep; drugs to wake and function, even if in a world of distortion and zombification. My peers were in a similar position. We were similar, yet dissimilar. Looking back now, I wonder how many of these young people were "sick" or were the symptoms displayed, a result of the powerful, mind altering constant medication. These drugs had changed me into someone (or, even, something) that not only I didn't recognise but my family and friends also didn't know.

I remember one horrific day, walking into the unlocked bathroom and seeing a young woman lying in a bath of ruby, red water, having slashed her wrists. I can't remember whether she survived or not.

So much of this time is a blur – my memories so confused. The drugs continually pumped in to me destroyed my ability to think or reason. I remember not wanting to see my parents – but can't remember exactly why. I didn't see them for weeks on end. I remember comfort eating and ballooning to a massive 12.5 stone and not "giving a damn". I know, in previous years, that was totally out of character. I was meticulous in my appearance. I now wore long baggy clothes and skirts to my ankles. I don't remember bathing or washing my hair. If I did attend to personal hygiene, it was only occasionally. I don't remember caring or anyone noticing. I do remember walking around the streets, late into the night with no set purpose or direction. How I never came to grief, I do not understand – God must have been there – somewhere. That area of

Manchester was notoriously dangerous –
prostitutes, pimps, drug dealers, gang fights. Yet,
physically I survived.

I remember, repeatedly, on these midnight jaunts,
self harming - either burning my hands and arms
with cigarette butts or cutting them with broken
glass or razors. I, usually, ended up at the local
Accident and Emergency Department. I became
"known" and often, as punishment, was stitched
without local anaesthetic but, somehow, I felt no
physical pain. This whole period – these years –
were a total period of numbness and unreality. I
lost total sense of time, of where I was and for
how long I was there and, even, who I was.

I know who I was told I was – bad, wicked,
attention seeking, worthless. I hated myself with a
vehemence, I had for life and humanity in general.

Even now, I get scared when I roll back time. This
is probably why it's something I rarely do and I
can't understand why I'm revisiting the past now.
This was not me. This is not the "me" I know now.
Yet, the medical fraternity told me that this
despicable creature was definitely me. I think the
diagnosis made was some psychotic illness and
the medication was to fit the mental disorder. Yet,
in the light of where I now am (and it does feel
light, compared to these years of darkness) what
came first? The questionable illness that those in
power diagnosed and prescribed for, or did the

medication prescribed turn me into this horrific self-loathing creature?

Throughout all these years, my dystonia , then unacknowledged, unrecognised and seen as a symptom of my psychosis, was present. Somehow, under the influence of these powerful drugs, it didn't really matter any more. It was all a part of me, this loathsome, manic being. Drugs had taken away any embarrassment I might have had in my mid-teens.

Teenagers – a normal teenager (it had been drummed into me I was not) – live in perpetual embarrassment if they have a prominent pimple, or blush in the presence of a boy they might have feelings for. Why could my embarrassment and lack of confidence due to these hideous spasms, not have been accepted by those around me, as a normal phase of those difficult teenage years. These dystonic symptoms made me feel that I didn't blend or fit in with the normality of my peers and made me want to seek sanctuary in being alone and out of sight.

At 16 years old, I needed empathy, support, and unconditional positive regard from those around me and intellectual understanding from those clinicians who diagnosed and then chose to condemn because they had no answers. These are the people who made me into this psychotic entity now entering adulthood, full of hate and anger, at both self and humanity.

Chapter 4.

From this period on and for many ensuing years, the memory of my life is still hazy. I can remember some major events but the detail and the order in, which they occurred, are impossible to recall. Most of this time, I was still being prescribed "heavy duty", mind altering drugs – mainly on repeat prescription, seeing very little or either GP or Consultant. I feel much of this difficulty in memory recall was also due to further episodes of, what I consider, barbaric E.C.T. treatment.

I feel a great sadness in this because this type of memory loss is not selective – the good times, as well as the bad are eradicated. Sometimes, friends or family might mention something pleasant from the past, of which I have no recollection, - as if, I was never even present and I find this quite unnerving and scary. Often, I don't admit this lack of memory to them but just "go along with it", more for their sake than mine. I still have difficulty recalling events of recent years; people's names and faces.

Something that was positive over these years was that my dystonia improved and eventually went into remission. Again due to unpredictable memory, I cannot pin point a date.

Having researched into the condition recently, this does fit a pattern. Remission for some and usually for younger people can come about. It is rare and sometimes, after years of remission, it can re-occur, as in my case. There seems to be no neurological explanation for this, neither to the trigger for its return.

Life events, in my early to late 20's, were, looking back and straining for memory recall, varied. I undertook several training courses which, in my earlier years and feeling perhaps destined for University, seemed both insignificant, yet, for some reason, anxiety laden. Anxiety would manifest itself in feelings of lack of ability to succeed.

I gained minor qualifications in typing; book-keeping; hotel reception and business studies. In the latter, I gained the highest marks, that year, in the entire Scottish F.E. system and received an award at Glasgow University. In the other exams, I usually gained distinctions or credits. Yet, I never felt good enough and I never enjoyed the mundane work they qualified me to undertake. I kept thinking back to the School I attended, at the age of 12 years old and of where they expected their pupils to be at this point in their lives. I had no B.A., M.A., no B.Sc or Doctorate, no piece of paper – the most important one it seemed to me - to tell me I was a success in my life.

After the tribulation around my G.C.E. examinations, the imminent psychiatrists had warned my parents that for me to strive for anything of too high an academic standing - over-taxing myself - might only lead to future psychological deterioration.

They were the experts. My parents believed them and more pertinently, I believed them, with every fibre of my being. I held on to this, year after year and each time I began a training course, that fear loomed and took hold of me. Usually, at this point, I would convince myself, particularly before any exam, that I might have another break-down. So off I'd go to the GP, encouraged by those around me and the pill-popping would begin, as also the repeat prescriptions which went on "ad infinitum" – valium, mogadon, even lithium. So the pattern carried on and my drug tolerance increased.

One of the most unhappy incidents, at that time in my life, was in connection with a relationship which further shattered my belief in self and mankind, in general. I began dating a young man , having been introduced to him by an elder cousin. John and I dated for 2 years - 2 reasonably happy years. Although, I felt I loved him (though, now, I suspect I didn't really know what love was) we came against friction outside of our relationship. John was Roman Catholic whereas I, at the time, was loosely Anglican. When John and I announced our engagement, we met much opposition - both from his priest and his mother. As I became better acquainted with his mother, by whom John was immensely influenced, her mood began to soften. However, the priest was very much against our union and the suggestion that both Anglican and Catholic priests, should come together in formulating a service that might satisfy both parties, was not a compromise he would make. Even, at this point, he made me sign a statement to the effect, that, if we did have children, they would be brought up as Roman Catholics.

We, eventually, did find a Roman Catholic priest, away from John's place of worship, who agreed to be involved in a wedding service of compromise. Everything then seemed to fall into place. The church was booked, the reception venue found and, eventually, invitations to guests sent out. I had chosen my wedding dress and those of my bride's maids.

Then, one evening, I received a heartbreaking phone call from John. He told me that he could not go through with the marriage. It was too complicated with us both being of different religious persuasion. I feel he had been greatly influenced by both his parish priest and his mother. At first, I couldn't comprehend the words he spoke. I had seen him earlier that day and there had been nothing of this nature discussed. I went into a paroxysm of tears, as he spoke to me. I think my main emotion was one of complete shock, similar to that of bereavement of someone very close. John wouldn't even answer some of my questions as to why he'd made this decision. In a cowardly way, he put the telephone receiver down and ended the conversation. When I tried to phone him back, his mother would not let me speak to him - protecting her "little boy".

My emotions were in turmoil. This had happened so unexpectedly, as far as I perceived and the wedding date was only 4 weeks away. I did a lot of crying and felt totally betrayed by someone I thought I loved and had trusted. I was also very hurt because I believed, strongly, that John loved me, reciprocally. I thought I knew this person I was about to marry but, now, it seemed I didn't really know him at all. I was also very angry, in the way in which he'd communicated his feelings to me, in that he couldn't tell me face to face. In all of this, it only spoke to me of my lack of self worth in that I had been rejected.

I was extremely emotional in response to this. Wouldn't most "normal" people have shared similar feelings? I was vocal in my emotion - tearful, angry, hurt, humiliated. Feelings such as this were fearful for my parents in my home setting, feeling that, perhaps, this would induce my former psychological symptoms.

They consulted my GP who arranged immediate admission for me to a nearby private hospital where I stayed for the next 7 days, until "I'd calmed down". I didn't need treatment - not that I received any, other than drugs to suppress my emotions. My mother did visit but I could sense the pain within her heart. I perceived, I had let my parents down again. I wanted someone to sit with me and listen to how I felt - to hug me, to make me feel special, in a way I now realised John did not feel about me. Yet, I couldn't expect or ask this from my mum and didn't feel I even deserved it. The Bad, Mad Girl I saw myself as.being, had resurfaced. Yet, I didn't feel ill. I just felt sad and very alone. I wanted the care and warmth of another human being, and, all I received were the inevitable drugs that calmed me down and pushed my true feelings further back into my personal black abyss. This period back in hospital, again (even though it was a general hospital) confirmed to me how the world viewed me - how I couldn't cope with life crises whether they be emotional or, as in years before, anything that brought about academic stress. My self-esteem was at an all time low. Whatever others believed of me, I believed also.

Chapter 5.

Skipping a number of years, in which I left my parental home and lived and worked away, life became somewhat chaotic. I'd missed my youth (late teens/early 20's) – going out with my peers – clubbing, shared holidays abroad – just being young, irresponsible and largely, carefree. Now, I was away from parental view and going to make up for it, in a big way! I suppose the expression was "going off the rails". I partied. I drank to excess. How I remained physically in tact, I do not know other than God must have had his covering hand on me. I acquired a battered MG Sports Car – the love of my life – and remember having races with other MG owners on a local by-pass, in the early hours of the morning, following nights of drinking to inebriation. I had no fears for my own safety, and still to my shame this day, no awareness for the safety of others.

I thought this style of life would make me happy, but all it did, was further convince me that I was despicable and more of a low-life than ever. My self-respect dropped to an all time low, as my alcohol and, prescribed, drug intake increased.

At some point, I again moved with regard to work, nearer home and began to see my parents a little more regularly. During this time, I met my earthbound (though, possibly, sent by the angels) redeemer who, within 2 years, became my husband. Over the years, pre our marriage, I told him bits of my history. I cared for him too much to pretend to be something I wasn't. Every time I told him a bit more, I expected him to go but, to my surprise, he didn't.

A year prior to our wedding, my father died. He'd been ill and deteriorating for a long time. Hence, my moving back nearer to the family home. At the time of his death, I was on holiday touring Europe with Rob. Knowing how ill he was, I made continual phone calls back home and each time, was assured of his physical stability. However, on my arrival home, I was informed my father had, in fact, died and been buried 2 days previously. I found it hard then in feelings and now in penning my emotional response to this. As before, my dear mother, in her distress, had consulted our GP as to how I would react on hearing the news. His advice was that I should not be called back home, that this would only cause extra grief to my family as a whole. When the news was broken to me, on my return - a horrendous ordeal for my darling mum - I was filled with consuming anger for this medical practitioner, an anger greater than anything I'd ever experienced to that date or since - a personal, frightening rage that engulfed me to my core.

Why, had this man denied me the chance to say "good bye" to my own father and grieve with my family at his funeral? Why was my involvement in the conclusion of his life and our relationship denied? I couldn't place blame or express anger to my family, they, once again, had deferred to professional advice and acted, as they felt, out of my best interests. Their grief at this time, was also, in retrospect, so great that my presence might have only compounded the intensity of this.

After visiting the grave as proof of finality, the shock; the anger; the sorrow; the enormity of what had happened; came upon me, in waves of no particular order. However, I came to an uneasy decision, this being that perhaps my exclusion from my father's funeral was in the family's greater interest. After all, I was unstable, of little use or value. I would have only made it worse for my mother and my sister.

Thank you, God, for by dear Rob. Initially, I took some of the anger I felt towards myself and, in self pity, as to "who I was" , out on him and we nearly parted. He let me lean on him. Yet he also built me up which, often I felt others   seldom did - not with the "Hadn't you better go to the GP and get the valium", doctrine but he built me up by his physical presence and the words he spoke to me, which meant so much. I began to sense, he believed in me as a person, as an adult which, even at the age of 26, I'd rarely felt or been allowed to feel. Something began to feel different and it was good.

Many years later, in fact last summer, (now my family see me more as an adult) my sister shared that at my father's funeral, tears had been pricking her eyes, yet, she had felt unable to let herself grieve publically . I felt a great sadness as she expressed this to me. Because of my recent emotional growth; because of my training and life circumstances; I know the relief and the positive therapy of tears. It's not weakness, whether from male or female, it's natural. It's normal. It's healing. Why do people feel it necessary to hide natural feelings such as these in similar circumstances? You can't push them down; lock them up; put them into a dark, deep cupboard. Do they come to you when you're alone, at the dead of night, when the whole world (save you) are asleep? My sadness, now I've grown, emotionally and spiritually – an adult, yet, can still choose to be a free child - is with you who choose to internalise something as great and all consuming as this. Others may choose to disagree with me and I do not deny anyone this right. These are MY feelings and equate also to my training and role in life, in the here and now.

If I'd only understood this all those years ago, when it was so important for me and my emotional survival.

My dear Rob and I did marry and the first years of marriage were not easy for either of us. The adjustment from being single to one of a couple was difficult but we coped. He was my rock and my GP visits   for my magic coping pills, became less.

Then, in both a joyous and, for me alarming event, little Lizzie entered the world and changed the shape of it, once again. Initial ecstasy and the pure wonderment of this creation, heaven sent, formed from combined genes, emotions and intellect, gave way to exhaustion of sleepless nights and 24 hour a day care. Reality dawned that no matter how wondrous and endearing this little baby was, the responsibility that came in this tiny bundle, was there for life. Life would never be the same.

Many of my old fears came back as to whether I could cope with this all-consuming responsibility. Words from those I'd considered of higher intellect or wiser than self - Doctors, Consultants, C.P.N, resounded in my head and I convinced myself, as per pattern of my life, I would fail.

I wasn't a good mother in those early days. I felt trapped, confined, resentful of this baby who'd interrupted the routine into which I was finally relaxing in days of early marriage. I couldn't cope with the new routine. I found it all fear consuming. I sometimes hated this child who had   taken over my life and taken away the peace of mind, I had just begun to feel, in my life with Rob. She didn't sleep or feed well.   She was edgy, tetchy, especially when we were alone together. I know,

now, I was communicating my feelings to her and this was her response.

This poor, beautiful and, I now know, perfect baby. At times, in my confusion of feelings and lack of self-under standing, I loved her so much that my heart literally ached yet I was also consumed with guilt and self- loathing. Why did I find the confines of motherhood so difficult? Was it because I, at the age of 28, was still that emotional child myself A child of adult appearance to the external world. Yet, a crying emotionally stunted and fearful child within?

I felt such inward guilt and shame, that it had been so easy for me to conceive when other couples try year upon year for children to no avail, yet, motherhood and all its confining aspects, threatened and terrified me .

Over a period of years, due to my felt sense of failure as a young mother and inability to cope, the pills did come back into my life, also periods of hospitalisation. The blur from E.C.T., toxic and powerful drugs again make this period or its length, hard to remember. One night medicated and having intoxicated myself to the point of numbness, I did take an overdose and was rushed by ambulance to an A & E Department.

I think this was more of a cry for help than a serious attempt to bring an end to my life. Somewhere in some part of my head was a sanity, which told me that I had responsibilities other than to self – to husband and more especially to daughter.

This again fills me with deep shame and those who attended me, patched the "physical bits" up and sent me out, again, into the reality of my world continually heaped the condemnation on.

How, my darling Rob stood by me, I will never understand. God created him especially for me. Rob could always manage to see something of worth in me - something of potential which others never seemed able to. I don't know whether he always gave me, unconditional positive regard .I don't think even a saint could have done that! I know, in retrospect and in shame, I took him to the limits – the arguments, me disappearing for hours on end. I remember once, "high" on medication, trying to jump from a moving car and him hitting me across the face. Other than that, he never (though sorely provoked) hurt me in any way. He was and is a wonderful, caring man and I cherish him with my whole heart and being. He is the one, who always had faith in me. When others walked away, he remained constant and close.

And as to that tiny young babe, she too has survived. In the very early days, more due to the efforts of Rob than myself. She is now a beautiful, young lady blossoming into adulthood who I also love with all my heart. Yes, we as a family, have our rows over normal everyday matters. How long she can stay out to; how far can she push us in getting her own way; massive telephone bills; too much make-up; skirts too short – but we have a normality, a sanity and hopefully, a sense of security in our home. We do row (name me a family with teenage children that doesn't !) but we also make-up. Someone apologizes and in this we show our love and support for one another, in both the good and bad times.

Chapter 6.

Perhaps, now, I need to describe how we, as a family, yet, mainly me – in change, have reached some state of normality and for most of the time, peace.

On admission to a modern/more enlightened psychiatric unit, 8 years ago, a credible diagnosis was made to my "illicit affair" with prescription drugs and, latterly, alcohol.

Whenever, from the age of 16 (initially through my dystonia being mis-diagnosed as a nervous breakdown) I thought I'd met a life situation that was too stressful, too anxiety ridden, my response would be flight from the situation - flight usually into mind numbing chemicals. I'd reach for the miracle potion that would relax and relieve me of this anxiety. I was actively encouraged to do this by both family and G.P., for THEIR fear of my response, if I didn't.

Up until the age of 16, I had never taken a "mood altering" (as they are now known) pill in any form. But when doctors baffled in medical diagnosis at my peculiar neck and head contortions and subsequent lack of self- confidence, they homed in on the psychological and prescribed me the likes of valium and their associated family. This began my journey – my hateful, dark, all consuming, self-reliance taking journey on whose black magic carpet I rode for over 20 years. These physicians drummed into me, concepts of me being a weak and inadequate, even "bad child" for portraying such attention seeking symptoms. They inferred it <u>was</u> possible for me to stop. When I, initially, cried out, in denial of this, in a small voice (that became smaller in defence, in the ensuing years of late teens) I was deemed irrational and divisive – a theory I believed also, in awe of those who knew "better." Hence, the medication increased. The small voice of protest, as to my powerlessness in these spasms, grew smaller and eventually disappeared. This voice disappeared, at the same time as Pauline, the flesh and blood person, disappeared also.

I was treated as Pauline, the ? psychotic, and so I took on the identity of that person. The more the drugs increased – the stronger they became – the less I cared about my life or the lives of those around me. But also in this, the more the medication robbed me of any fight or energy, the more malleable I became and "they" were happy – their diagnosis confirmed.
This pattern, as described, continued, year upon year with small patches of lucidity when I felt safe enough to decrease my pills.

Yet a point ,to be my saving grace, though not seen as this at the time was when the medical profession, in general, became more enlightened in the area of drug dependency. They became more aware of the addictive nature (in the same way as cocaine or heroine) that drugs such as diazepam could be and how tolerant the body can become after long term usage, needing greater amounts to create the same psychological effect. Hence, my GP refused to prescribe me any more. I'm sure it must have been a "weaning off" process, rather than complete withdrawal, due to the dangers of such a radical cessation. Whatever, it was, I was filled with terror that my "life coping mechanism" was being taken from me.

So, then began the introduction of alcohol usage in my life coping strategy. I say usage rather than consumption because that is how I "used" it. Many people can drink socially with no ill effect, other than perhaps a mild hangover in the morning. I "used" alcohol to give me confidence – to socialise; to do the weekly shopping; to survive and numb the fear I had of engaging in every day normal life. If I didn't drink, I'd "use" strong painkillers (codeine) bought over the counter at the chemist. Addicts, as that is what I finally accepted I was are incredibly devious and very deceitful. I'd hide alcohol and pills all around the house. I'd travel great distances to purchase my codeine at various different pharmacies. I'd lie and cheat to preserve my "life-giving cache".

As unobvious as it was to me, it was most obvious to my GP and Rob that my life was becoming out of control and I was admitted to an

A.T.P. (Addiction Therapy Programme) unit in a private psychiatric hospital.

This was to be my life-saver - physically, psychologically and spiritually. Again, I thank God that we did have private medical cover that provided for my treatment – so many addicts/victims of life do not and this grieves me greatly. THIS has given me that burning desire, over the past years, to reach and help these people, less fortunate than I was, yet, equally needy.

I remained on the ATP unit, as an in-patient, for 12 weeks. Initially, I hated it and I felt very scared. They wanted me to cope outside, in the real world, without my drug of choice. This had been my coping device, for so many years, in a fearful environment where I felt I had few places of safety! Impossible!

For many days, I refused to even leave my room. There were 'one to one' sessions with counselors but mainly the "work" was done in groups – male and female together.

I think what eventually touched me, was that all the counselors had been former addicts themselves – alcohol, drugs, gamblers. They had, even if years before, "worn" my shoes, maybe felt my fear. They were credible examples of life after addiction.

After further time, I even began to benefit from group sessions. It was fine and infect desired, just to be yourself - no facades, no masks. You could be honest about your feelings – in the past and the here and now. Unless you were honest, you were possibly destined for failure and relapse.

It was hard – very hard, at times and some patients (those who gave up because of this, and returned to their lives of addiction) didn't finish the programme. Some of these have since died or are heading in that inevitable direction.

We did have to admit to our addiction and as part of our treatment, had to attend external AA or NA (Narcotics Anonymous) meetings. This prospect, initially, abhorred me. Who would be at these – tramps, winos, and homeless vagrants? Yes, there were these people (usually the ones who continued to "use") but there were also doctors, dentists, lawyers, nurses and housewives. I learnt addiction does not discriminate and unless you can admit to your addiction and abstain whether lawyer or vagrant, you will never recover.

These 12 weeks at this hospital changed my life – a phrase sometimes used – "changed it beyond my wildest dreams".

I can't blame my distain misdiagnosis for my fall into addiction. Perhaps there was a genetic tendency for this already in place at birth. But I feel I can blame the treatment of being prescribed powerful, mood-altering drugs at an early age and being diagnosed with a psychological rather than biological illness, for some of this. I do look back sometimes and feel sad at the shape and form my life had taken as a consequence. But, I know I can only live in the here and now, or else will become consumed with anger and resentment. Not a safe place for me to be.

The programmed, the counsellors and my fellow "non using" addicts, taught me how to love and respect myself again. Had I ever done this? How I could be strong and cope with life, without my drug of choice?

Therapy, especially 'one to one', helped me to find out who I really was. I'd spent years in "blackout" as a result of powerful, mind-numbing drugs. I neither cared nor knew what my true identity was. I was encouraged to dig deep to rediscover the real Pauline. At times it was painful and I didn't like this – the ensuing tears and sadness. Yet, I feel I emerged a "whole" person – a person of worth and potential who felt it was, now, OK to openly express tears and anger, as well as laughter and happiness. I didn't have to cut bits of myself off (as learnt as a child) from the outside world and present only those "bits" I thought were acceptable. That feeling of being able to be true to self felt freeing, liberating and so good.

Chapter 7.

Leaving the ATP unit and rejoining the outside world was quite a fearful prospect for me but not, as in years before, when I'd felt institutionalized. I felt I was still growing emotionally and maturing but, now, I had acquired "tools" (STRONGER than medication) to manage my own life. At 40 years old, I was beginning to grow up and became an adult! Even though married and with my own child, I had never really felt this before and it was amazing and liberating.

I did, in this process of healing, feel God touch my life. Sometimes, I couldn't see him very clearly but I sense, in retrospect, that He was there, waiting for me to turn my eyes back to him. Christian friends (and Christian counsellors) had played their part too. The human face of Christianity and deeds enacted, meant more than someone just saying they were praying for me.

As a Pre or Young Christian and an addict, I was cynical, and words and deeds spoke volumes - more so than promises of prayer. Now, years on, my belief in prayer is far greater but I still feel Christianity needs a face and that actions speak louder than words, especially to those without or having little faith.

After two years post my hospital discharge, I was invited back to train as a peer-supporter – a credible intermediary between patient and counsellor. This in itself, for me, was a challenge and again an opportunity for personal growth and development.

After initial training, my role involved greeting and setting the scene for new patients; speaking on the phone to prospective or past patients and their families and also, working in Group Therapy with the trained counsellors.

I really enjoyed this role and it helped me to realize that I wanted to take this further. Would I have the capabilities, intellectual and psychological , to train to be a counsellor? I talked this through with staff members and was encouraged to apply for a counselling certificate course.

Again with initial trepidation, I applied to Salford University and even after disclosing my past history of addiction , was given a place on a one-year part-time course.

I looked forward to Thursday afternoons with a passion. I so loved what I was doing. It was basically a counselling skills course. We studied the theory of Carl Roger's, Person Centred Therapy. We practised on one another but not in role play. We used real life situations and so confidentiality was always to the fore. In personal development groups, in a similar way, we were encouraged to be real about ourselves. How could we possibly expect others (i.e. prospective clients) to "open-up" without experiencing that feeling of vulnerability from a personal perspective? To grow, we had to be vulnerable. Some students found this very difficult. Some decided the course was not for them. Not me. Like an excited child, I wanted more and more. I felt I had "come home". This was something I loved and wanted to take forward into my life. Others had helped me for such a long time. Now was my time to give back.

This course (although not a qualification to counsel "real" clients) was continually assessed – written assignments; logs kept on our own personal growth and development; and the dreaded one hour video-taped session of ourselves counselling another student. This was not only nerve wracking – the assessment of yourself as counsellor- but entailed many hours of academic work – preparing a verbatim transcript and then a critique on your role, in relation to theory.

I passed this certificate with distinction. Mainly, I feel due to my enthusiasm and increasing self-belief in my ability. But the Diploma was different, in my quavering thoughts. This was the pinnacle – the one that said you're "good enough" to work with real people, not merely students you chatted to over a coffee, in the canteen. Could I do this? Did I have the ability?

The interviewing panel obviously thought so, as they did allocate a place for me on the two year Diploma Course. Initially, and true to character at the first session, I met with students with 1st degrees, teachers, nurses, others with higher academic achievements than myself and my heart "slumped". How would I keep pace with them? The tears welled and I felt sick. Was this the end of the dream? Was this (medical practitioners' words, again, ringing in my ears) "too much for me?"

The old Pauline would have fled or found an excuse to leave. She most certainly would have "popped a pill" or got intoxicated, in a bid to alleviate anxiety. She would have done this for so long, then it still would have all "become too much" and she would have left. There would have been a valid excuse, used time over again, to leave jobs or adult education, "I'm suffering from stress – that's just me. I have to leave for fear of making myself sicker".

Although the employer/the tutor would have made understanding comments and, on the surface for me, it would have seemed the best and most sensible action to take, my self worth, my self-respect, would have plummeted and I would, once again, be fulfilling the messages given to me when I was 16. Messages from the physicians, my family – people who, I then thought, knew better and whose advice I should follow.

Yet, Pauline, now having a better understanding of self and capability, was in a more positive place, to make her own "adult" decision. Yes, I still was afraid I might fail academically, that I wouldn't have the confidence to counsel "real clients". Instead of hiding these fears away and them growing and distorting into something hideous and terrifying , instead of "fleeing" from the situation in the basic, pre-historic flight or fight syndrome, I chose to stay and face my anxiety. This was when the realisation dawned on me that I did have enough courage, self determination and personal confidence to "do this thing", without the need for a "confidence fix" of either pill or drink. What freedom! What liberty! What a life I now potentially had!

In the weekly Personal Development Groups, of 12 individuals who came to know one another so well – the positive and the negative – over these two years, I chose to share my feelings, my emotions, my fears. And, it was again, liberating - not people pleasing or saying what I thought others might want me to say or agree with. I stopped feeling like the chameleon of earlier years, who changes his true identity to blend and merge into his surroundings, nor did I censor what I chose to share. I felt proud to be an individual and to be able to express myself in this way. Students became very real in these Groups and the atmosphere wasn't always one of comfort. There was challenge in that room but with this there was also support. That was the purpose of those Groups. How could we, as counsellors, even begin to understand clients' fears or frailties, unless we understood and explored our own?

I was amazed at what others shared in this room – similar feelings of insecurity; fear of failure; unhappiness in their lives; shameful episodes from the past still haunting, in the present. The honesty in that room was incredible – something, sadly, missing very often, in the "real world", to the detriment of humanity.

Don't misunderstand and believe these were sessions of selfish confession for mass absolution from the Group, and they certainly were not personal therapy. Many tears were shed in that Group, sometimes of grief, sometimes of anger. It was no easy ride but something very special and very real was there. I know this was a secular course, (even though 6 out of 20 of us were Christians) but, at times, I could feel the healing presence of God. I believe there was some kind of spiritual covering for those who wanted to reach out and touch it.

In addition to this Group, each student had to attend 20 sessions with a qualified counsellor. This made great sense to me, because sometimes in the Group "boxes", having been locked tight for years, began to open and spill out. They needed further personal exploration, to be fully understood and maybe acted upon or laid to rest by students. Also, sometimes in listening to clients' issues, something personal to yourself (a similar situation or emotion) might arise, that you, as counsellor, needed to explore with your own therapist, before you could give of your best to the client.

So after five months of theory, assignments and practice on one another, under the tutor's watchful eye, those who were deemed "safe", were sent out into the real world of counselling. I - Pauline Pearce, was deemed "safe" to counsel in the Real World - amazing, beyond my wildest dreams!

My placement, for 18 months, was at a GP Practice, in quite a deprived area of Cheshire. I don't like that word so perhaps my explanation might be that there was high unemployment, high rates of vandalism, teenage pregnancy, domestic and street violence and drug abuse. This makes it sound like "hell on earth" and to many who lived there it probably was. Yet, the clients I worked with over those months, were the most lovely of people – depressed often, having relationship difficulties, suffering bereavement but, almost to each client I met and had the privilege to work with, I found the most warm-hearted and generous of individuals.

How sad, I feel, that the minority – the angry, the greedy, the destructive – can colour one's view of an area before it's experienced in totality. Another lesson, indeed, for me as counsellor.

I loved my work here. Again it felt this was so right for me, as an individual. I felt I had now got something I could give – that was in God's plan at my creation. I even felt that, perhaps, I did have to endure those dark years for what seemed like eternity, to give me the qualities and understanding I now needed to be involved in this work. In fact, I remember one balmy summer evening, sitting with friends, having shared a meal together, that I would never have believed I could be so happy. Happiness, in my life (prolonged happiness) had never seemed an option.

Chapter 8.

Yet, almost as soon as those words had tumbled from my lips, a part of my life began to change. It must have been several months later but those words, rang clear in my head and haunted me for weeks on end.

My head and neck started doing - all I can describe it as - unbidden movements. My head began to tilt slowly, almost imperceptibly to those who knew me, towards my right shoulder, giving me pain, and pins and needles down my arm. The passion of my life is horse riding, so after numerous falls at various stages of my riding career, I've been a regular attendee at the osteopath. I now presented myself there for numerous sessions. Nothing seemed to change or improve.

My next port of call was to the GP who, after I had visited so regularly over the "dark" period, I now had not seen for what seemed like years! He sent me off to the physiotherapist who put my, now painful, neck in traction, which caused, post-treatment, even more pain and numbness. Still, I persisted and was pushed higher up the echelon of seniority, in the phsyio department, as each individual failed to understand what was occurring in my skeletal frame.

During all this time, struggling with pain, neck spasm and now tremor, I continued my course and continued to see my clients. As my symptoms deteriorated and I found it harder to keep eye contact for long periods with them, I felt I needed to give some explanation. I didn't want my clients to think my fidgeting in the chair was due to boredom in their presence. Nor, that they might make any negative assumptions of their own that might affect our relationship and consequently, the quality of our work together. I just gave a brief, hopefully (to them – certainly, not to me) re-assurance that I had a "problem" with my neck and that it was being treated. I also gave each client the option of seeing another counsellor, if my fidgeting etc. was "off-putting". Thankfully, none chose to do so. I also checked with my supervisor was I right in continuing to see clients? I didn't want my problem to adversely affect my work. She was re-assuring in that the course of action I had taken in minimalist disclosure about self and then turning the whole focus of the session from me to them , was fine.

I began, after six or so months, to get very worried. It had taken a long time for my memory to regress back to 1972, when I was 16 years old with similar symptoms. I think I sub-consciously did not want to "take" myself there. But, now, all physical treatment failing to improve my condition, I was "there" again in that horrible, scary place – yet, now, I was an adult, with adult emotion.

I tried to be logical but couldn't understand (as the now, attending medics) what was happening. Dear God, and I said this in the form of prayer and not name taken in vane, was I having a nervous break-down?

Were the psychiatric fraternity, of the past, right in their original diagnosis? Had I striven beyond my psychological and academic capabilities? Was I weak and frail in mind? God, where were you? Where were the answers? I had thought I'd really grown and matured as an individual, over the past years. But had I?

So many factors did not weigh up in relation to former circumstances. Was I stressed as this was an exacting and demanding course, both academically and emotionally, especially when listening to the pain of others?

One has to learn early on as a counsellor that you cannot cure the "ills of the world", and you cannot become too emotionally and personally involved. You have to keep yourself "safe". This might sound cold-hearted but is not meant to be. You can be totally with the client, for that one hour. You can listen and respond empathically. You can, at times, even cry with them. But you, as much as you may wish, cannot be a miracle worker. God is the only one - in my belief - who can choose to do this. You, as a counsellor, are certainly not that! But, you can be there with and for them - to listen, to support in a way that they have perhaps never experienced before. You don't give them answers to their problems - as so many people think - but you can support them, in finding their own solutions. The positive impact on a client doing this for himself, with the counsellor alongside, creates a far greater and lasting impact for him than if you told him how to put his life in order - if, indeed, you were ever to assume you did have the answers. Fake or impostor counsellors - and, unfortunately, there are some of these about - might claim to have these answers but these are dangerous, reckless charlatans who can wreck the lives of those at their most vulnerable.

Counsellors, sincere and caring counsellors, can help their clients grow and eventually and hopefully, become independent - able to find their own solutions from within. The aim of all counselling, is to help that client to grow and mature, to become more self-reliant and self-resourceful. If the client's dependence on the counsellor becomes too great, power and self-reliance can be taken from him, placing it on the counsellor as the expert/ professional with all the answers. This is the way I viewed the "experts" who attended me, in my teenage years and this took me further into feelings of dis-belief in self and my capability to cope in that "big, bad world".

This is the philosophy of Carl Rogers, the pioneer of Person Centred Counselling, and I believe in it, with passion, from both personal experience and

from working with clients and watching them grow and develop into mature and capable individuals.
At times, in my work, I did feel a level of stress - feelings of wanting to do more for a particular client, but I didn't feel burnt out because I had given more than I had or more than I should. I could, most times, leave this stress behind, in the counselling room.

If a counsellor gives too much   to a particular client, what has she left to give to her remaining clients,   with equally difficult life situations and anxieties?   This has to be monitored by both counsellor and supervisor,   in order for the therapist, to give of her best and equally to all. It is also acts as a personal,   psychological health check for the counsellor. I felt I had done this, in a way to keep myself safe and to be able to function well, in my role as therapist

Yet,   could I,   with these strange physical symptoms, be heading for burn-out? I, certainly, did not feel this. I felt great compassion for each of my clients and a sense of wanting to wave the "fairy god-mother's magic wand"   to make everything better, but I knew the unreality of this. I enjoyed the positive stress of this work (both academic and in therapy sessions) - the privilege of trying to help a client make positive changes in his life, if that was needed and to bring better quality into his life, whatever the circumstances. Sometimes clients made great progress   and made life-changing decisions in a very positive way. Other times, the client would just sit and share the enormity and sadness of a life from which there seemed no "escape route" but, even then, they admitted something positive came from this. The fact that someone else wanted to listen, to empathise and show care towards them. For one hour, each week, that burden was "dumped" and released, and they left a little lighter.

I loved this work. I gained, personally, so much from what I was doing and, hopefully, the difference (even if small) I could make for others. Yet, why was I manifesting symptoms, at this moment in time, that I'd experienced in 1972? Symptoms that told me I was, perhaps, becoming psychologically unwell? I did not feel like this inside my head or in my emotions. But, could I trust my feelings?

During this period of time, I had a cancer scare and had investigations, leading to a minor operation, to determine whether I, indeed, did have cervical cancer. To my already anxious mind, this was, somehow, a secondary concern and almost cast aside. My husband and daughter worried far more, as we awaited the results of the tests. To me, in my intense confusion, at this time, I almost wanted it to be cancer. At least then, I could die an honourable death, rather than be labelled psychologically ill or attention seeking, again. I think in this I had momentary insanity, in my fear and confusion, caused by these other symptoms. Fortunately, my sane head later returning, and receiving the "all clear", I was incredibly thankful and gave my prayers of thanks to God.

I think my saving grace in all of this, was when I saw the Senior Physiotherapist. I have described my ascension up the ranks of physio seniority, in THEIR confusion also. This time, it worked to my benefit.

This woman, immediately noticed some miscorrelation in my neck and spine vertebrae, and a difference of level in my scapulas which to her, in her knowledgeable position, spoke volumes. She centred on my neck and head tremor also and the terminology of "Parkinson's" was mentioned. This did concern me but, even in this, there was some relief that she believed there was a physical cause.

Accordingly, I was referred to a Consultant Neurologist - not, as I had dreaded for many months, to a psychiatrist. After many neurological tests, he gave me a diagnosis, that same day. I could hardly take his words in. There WAS some authentic, medical terminology for these peculiar symptoms! This meant others before, others now, suffered the same muscular spasms and tremors. I felt, somehow, some form of elation. This man had confirmed to me, and to the world, that I was a sane human being.

However, some time later, as he continued to inform me of the nature of dystonia, I lost some of this euphoric feeling. I asked many questions, which he patiently answered. (This was a private consultation!) Yet, some of these responses were not those I wanted to hear but knew I must. He said the way this condition had manifested itself in me, as a teenager and then gone into remission several years later, was quite typical of its course. However, the older you were, when it returned, the less chance there was of further remission.

He said that my dystonia appeared mainly focal (head, neck, occasional voice tremor). I asked hard questions and he gave me hard and true answers. I needed to know the full facts. I asked would the dystonia remain static or could it spread to other parts of the body. He admitted he didn't really know because it affects each individual sufferer, in an individual way. But, he didn't exclude the possibility of it spreading.

Dr Enevoldson said it was a difficult condition to treat and again, different sufferers responded in varying way to treatment. In great honesty, he said drug therapy could help some patients but often, the high level of drugs needed to bring about improvement, could leave the sufferer practically comatose. There was surgery but any brain surgery had its dangers and was usually a last resort. The best option, in his opinion, was for me to have regular injections, into the affected muscles, of a derivative of Botulin Toxin. Bot Tox in its rawest form is a deadly poison that paralyses its "victim" but this derivative, in its weaker form, worked by intercepting (i.e. paralysing) messages from brain to the affected muscle/s and, hopefully, controlling unbidden movement.

He did stress that this treatment did not work for everyone and, if it did, it took some time to gauge how strong the dose needed to be and into which exact muscles the injections should be administered. There also were potential side-effects - one of the most common, for the first few weeks after treatment, difficulty in swallowing. What Dr Enevoldson was telling me was, "There is no cure for this condition but, maybe, we can help you control some of the symptoms".

He told me that Private Health Companies would not finance this treatment, due to its expense and that the NHS waiting list for Bot-tox treatment was long. If I was interested in taking this way forward, he would add my name to this list, via his colleague Dr Moore. What could I lose? I could only, hopefully, gain so I agreed to this course of treatment.

I left that consultation rather dazed. A part of me felt such relief that this was a recognised medical condition. Yet, another part of me, slowly began to realise I might remain with these strange contortions and tremors until, maybe, my life's end.

Chapter 9.

My life style, at present, would have to change and was already changing. I was in so much pain, at this point, that I could only walk very short distances - from house to car. I hadn't ridden a horse for many months and this had always been my way of finding time out for self, from the stresses of life. I couldn't drive the car or even travel far, as a passenger, due to searing pain caused by every bump or lump in the tarmac. My life (my comparatively newly found life) had been one I greatly enjoyed and was one of physical activity - long walks with Robin and friends, horse riding, swimming, cycling. All of these, I now could not continue with and I felt, because of this, there was a great vacuum in my life. Yet, I could still be useful in the fact that I could counsel, and my University course and client work became very important to me.

I visited my GP for advice - mainly in connection with pain relief. He had never heard of dystonia and although I handed him an informative leaflet, I felt he showed little interest or desire to become better informed or to understand its implications on a sufferer.

I told him how much my counselling course and my client work meant to me but, how difficult re; the pain factor, both the travelling to University or sitting still with a client was. I told him how the course, the friendship with other students, seeing my clients was now, very much a part of my quality of life as so many other areas were becoming excluded, due to my physical limitations. I was also, two thirds of the way through my year two of Diploma studies - assignments up to date; assessments passed; the required client hours nearing target. I wanted, and needed, to continue. Could he help me in any way, whilst I was waiting for my Bot-tox clinic appointment to come through?

His response was ironic and so un-empathic as to be, at this point, laughable. "Why do you have to put yourself through this unnecessary physical pain? It's ludicrous travelling 40 miles each week to the university, when car journeys are so painful for you and why add to this stress, by trying (and I feel he said this in irony) to "help" other people? Sometimes, people have to change life-plans and it can't be avoided. Why can't you?"

My anger at this was intense. This was my life he was attempting to "re-arrange" and take control away from me - or that's how I felt. Maybe, these were only words but, years before, when I had felt intimidated by physicians such as this GP, I would have listened and acted upon their suggestions. I had always thought people, in authority such as this, knew what was best for me, so poor was my self-belief and confidence.

I told him, now, in no uncertain terms, that I chose to continue my studies to their completion. It was difficult biting back the tears at his lack of understanding and him "writing me off" as others had before. I wanted, so much, for him to see a new strength in me. But, in other ways, what did it matter if he chose to see the "old" rather than the "new" me? I knew I'd changed, for the positive, even if he didn't.

Years before, this would have been a wonderful excuse for the old Pauline to take the easy option when "the going got hard". But not now. It made me want to fight harder to achieve my aim, which began as a small seed years before and had grown and matured, as had I. My GP's next response to me, and to what I feel he perceived as an uncooperative attitude, was to suggest valium might help control some of the pain and spasm. He wanted to make out a prescription for this - the very drug that began my long and dark journey into addiction, at the age of 16. I could hardly believe his words. Had he forgotten my history , so soon? Did he know nothing of addiction? Years before I would have been deliriously happy to be given these pills so easily. Today, the mention of their name and any connection of my accessibility to them, terrified me.

I left the surgery confused, bewildered and very angry but with a determination to carry on with my training and work regardless.

I, due to the course requirements, have an amazing personal therapist, Kate, who has been my "life-saver" during these confusing months. Kate has M.S. and I feel is in a far worse physical place than myself. Plus, she has been a sufferer for many long years. She is a very brave lady and I "love her to bits". When I visit Kate, I mainly offload my burden on her. On this occasion, it was anger at my GP's response and I find, having this space for self, immensely helpful. She, partly because of her illness and fight she has had as a consequence of this, has been my inspiration. She, jokingly, says that she will be counselling clients on her death bed and I almost believe this!

Kate, too, is a Person-Centred Counsellor, with other eclectic skills used where appropriate. This is a similar place, in practical experience, I would like to reach, over the next few years. Although, highly experienced and skilled, she still does not give me the answers but she makes me, by her attendance - her intensity with me - feel very special, valued and confident in control of my own life. The answers I have found, from within myself, during these sessions have been incredible - some life-changing and they have given me so much strength - strength to beat the emotional damage of this illness and find new quality in my life. After much soul searching and thought, as a result of one of these sessions, I did find some compromise with regard to the valium.

In order to cope with the physical pain involved in car journeys, I began - whilst waiting for my hospital appointment to arrive - to take the tablets on an irregular basis (not as prescribed, 3 times a day) I gave them over to the charge of my husband to administer to me, as needed. This stopped me feeling so fearful with them being in the house. This might sound childlike but I have a healthy fear of valium, which I feel is good. If I lost this, I would be concerned.

I found ways of sitting at University lectures to minimise my head tremor and pain. I used a chair, with a swinging desk top, on which I would pile cushions brought from home. I would rest my head on the palm of alternative hands. Too much leaning on one arm, brought on pins and needles. This physical support helped me to control my head tremor. Tutors and students had been very tolerant of me, moving around during lectures, as this helped too much stiffness and pain setting in.

My problems did not seem to affect my counselling work too dramatically – though sometimes sitting still for an hour was a little difficult. I always told each new client, on their first visit, why I sat a little strangely – learning on cushions on my lap or desk surface. Sometimes they might ask why, and I would give a brief answer but I always stressed that this time was for them and not about me.   I didn't want them minimising their problems or censoring anything they might wish to disclose, because of MY "physical problems". As far as I was aware, once I had shared my "bit", the counselling sessions took on a normality akin to those before my condition had set in.

Since, my first Bot-tox injection, I have had much relief from pain, which was a miracle in itself. Also, my head tremor became less severe. I began to be able to walk a lot further and also returned to horse-riding – though not at the level I rode 12 months ago. I'm starting to feel a lot more normal and also (most times) more accepting of my condition – certainly less fearful of the future. I have learnt to live a day at a time. If one day is particularly bad, more often than not, emotionally or physically, the next is better.

The further away I am from the next Bot-tox treatment, the more troublesome the symptoms become. I've had 2 treatments, to date, and am a fortnight away from the third. At present, the tremor and spasms are more pronounced. But, and this is were I am eternally grateful, the searing pain I endured pre treatment, has not returned. I thank God, daily, for this. Also, I do now have stronger belief that the Bot-tox will eventually, give me greater relief as the dosage and areas into which it is injected, are found. I have to come to terms with this being a long and, possibly, unpredictable process. I need to be patient and this is NOT one of my virtues! I, also, too have to come to terms that, possibly, these physical symptoms may not get much better.

With so many questions re my physical health, it is imperative I look to God for peace in acceptance, whatever the future may bring.

Chapter 10.

Now in my home domain, and remembering that day on holiday in August 2001, when I began looking back into my thoughts/ feelings, I felt a negativity in attitude to my life and a fear of the future. I don't know quite why I chose to put pen to paper. I don't know why I decided to look back into painful episodes which I'd avoided thinking about for many years. The result of this has been immensely cathartic and positive for me. I, now, feel on track and able to see the future, in a far more positive light.

I still, as hard as I try not to, suffer from embarrassment when, for example, walking in busy areas and I know eyes are upon me – my head in some bizarre contortion. It doesn't concern me with friends or people who know about my condition. They know I look and walk a bit differently, but that my brain, my intellect and capabilities are still intact.

I think because I was "labelled" psychologically disturbed, when I was a teenager, it comes into my mind – though I try hard to ignore it – that people, who don't know me, might label me as this now, observing my strange spasms. I often , in defence of this and to try and be a bit braver, go out of my way to make sensible conversation with people in shops, on trains etc. This is my way of coping with possible stigmatisation which I abhor in any form, by and towards anyone, in this, sometimes, cruel world.

However, I think in the whole episode of my life and after my diagnosis 10 months ago, the biggest challenge for me, has been to accept the course my life has taken and how different my path might have been, if I had been diagnosed accurately in 1972.

For some reason, it took many months before this impacted on me. Yet, when it finally did, my emotions took an enormous "battering".

I, because of being mis-diagnosed in my teenage, formative years (and I feel the adjective "formative" is crucial in this) had absolutely no idea "who" I was. Teenage years, by their very nature, can be a very confusing time for any young person. You are neither adult nor child. You are searching for your own personal identity and character – separating from peers with whom only, so recently, you almost wanted to be "cloned" with - to blend or merge with, to be one of the accepted crowd. Yet, now, adulthood approaching and separation from peers naturally occurring, you have to find your own very special and individual identity. A difficult time for the most well balanced young person.

At 16 my focus, was to succeed academically, with future expectations of attending university, leading to a creditable career. Then, possibly, marriage and motherhood.

Yet, as if by cruel fate, all this was snatched away, in what seemed like an instant from me, by medical misdiagnosis. My life, as I knew it and expected it to be, ended there and my future became both a mystery and, even, insignificant to me.

I did not know who I was. I had no identity other than the labels those physicians placed upon me – psychotic; attention seeking; wicked to cause everyone so much trouble. And, in my haze of powerful medication, I believed them and often acted the part they expected me to. I felt a failure - a detestable and unloved entity. In fact, I felt de-humanised and my faith in self and humanity was at its lowest ebb.

As described and as the years progressed, I, in my own eyes, continued to fail and the self-loathing increased. Yet my darling Rob (who I still believe was God sent) began the long journey we took together, back to sanity and peace. I feel God especially sent him so that we could help one another in this life. Rob is deaf (total loss of hearing in one ear, 30% hearing in the other) and we have, mutually, aided one another these past 18 years. Although, managing reasonably well at work, social events can sometimes be a nightmare for him – background noise or music, others speaking loudly – can make a situation, which we would often avoid, very difficult. Now, he is more confident, socially, because I can be there to repeat lost words in conversation and ensure he knows what is generally going on around him. Rob has, at times, been quite depressed over the years, especially after a further significant loss of hearing eight years ago, with a realisation that, possibly, as he gets older, this loss may continue. Robin suffers from stigmatisation too when, for example, a shop assistant unable to get a response from him due to his poor hearing, makes some caustic comment. He has learnt, over the years, to become less affected by this. He knows he is not stupid or lacking in intelligence, even if she/he doesn't appreciate the fact. I, with my strange neck spasms, have learnt from his attitude too – though it is still early days for me!

God did bring us together I'm sure of that now – to support and care for one another in what can sometimes be a very cruel world. People are so often judged at face value – their physical appearance; the clothes they wear; the area in which they live, being held of prime importance. Why are we, as human beings - God's creations and I'm sure he did create us all for some special reason - often so unkind to one another? God also saved Robin and I from being two lonely people apart when he brought us together. Two people, a little different perhaps, a little set apart from others because of our differences, but to Him, two very special and loved people. His hand covered us. and continues to do so.

What has helped me in, gradual, acceptance of dystonia are a number of factors. I do believe in the healing God - even though, I've lost sight of him many times over the past 12 months. Yet, I know others may not. I might be asked "If your God is so good, so great, then why doesn't he heal you?" My answer is that I don't know. But I can hold on to the fact that one day I will know why. And that reason will be for good and not for evil.

Certainly, this illness has made me feel more compassionately for others, in many different situations. I feel even more determined that I want to work as a counsellor, to help others find the best quality possible in their lives, despite their circumstances, and in my work and to this date, I have seen this come about.

My own healing began when I started to understand me - the real me - in a better way. I didn't accept any more who other people told me I was. It was life-changing , life saving even, to begin to know how to reach for those answers myself. Sometimes I didn't like what I found. Other times I did, and could actually tell myself that I really was quite a nice person. I don't think I had ever really believed that, even as a child.

My three years studying counselling gave me further insight into my own identity and also the skill to help others find theirs. Sometimes, individuals, in a cursory way, feel they do know "who they are" but, then, some life challenge (illness, bereavement) may come about and this outwardly strong person, may begin to crumble and lose that self they thought they knew and understood. How often, unless sometimes forced in some negative sense, do we get that chance or time, just to stand back and truly look into ourselves – to find and accept that inner person – both the good and the bad?

I feel that unless I'd had that opportunity to look inward, to grow and mature as an addict in recovery; as a trainee counsellor and with my own counsellor; the difficulties I'd have had in coping with this new chapter in my life (dystonia) would have been overwhelming.

I'm not saying, especially before, and when, I first received my diagnosis, I was not distraught. The tears I have shed, at losing parts of my old life, have been copious. It has not, and is still not, easy.

I don't experience the same quality of life as I did before but I have an equivalent, if different, one and it feels good – often, more than good!! Many times, illness can also give you something special that unless you've had this experience from the inside, you can't understand. Perhaps it's something to do with life feeling, suddenly, more intense; more valuable and needing to be lived to the full. But,   without acceptance of new limitations how can this come about?

Illness, especially I feel chronic illness, is difficult to accept, particularly as you become older in years. If it brings disablement – either physical or psychological – it can feel as if life itself has ended or that, because quality of life is so poor then, there is nothing "out there" that can possibly bring any joy or hope again. To dramatise perhaps to the extreme maybe similar   to surviving   - certainly not living - from day to day, waiting for the release of death.

I'm not saying that's what it is like for sufferers of dystonia, who don't cope well,   emotionally or spiritually, with their illness. When I initially met, the first dystonia sufferer - other than self - at the   Bot-tox clinic, I so wanted to see people affected by this,   looking as if they were living reasonably "normal" and contented lives.

Perhaps, I chose a bad day. There were only two ladies there, both displaying similar symptoms to myself. I really needed to talk to them. I needed some reassurance that life could become reasonably "normal", as to this point, I had felt very isolated. Initially, because I had never met a dystonia sufferer and also because my GP (and the GPs at the practice where I counselled) had never encountered this condition either.   I felt somewhat of an oddity and needed a feeling of connection to somebody or something.

As these ladies spoke and I listened, they described how (and they were both long-term sufferers) dystonia had devastated their lives. This came mainly from their embarrassment at the way people outside viewed them; how these ladies felt they were judged at face value.

One lady said she rarely left her house, only and occasionally, in the safety of her husband's company. The other said she no longer attended any social events, even family gatherings, as she couldn't bare people (relations, past close-friends) seeing how grotesque she now looked. They both said they were virtually "house-bound". They both looked immensely distressed.

This was not what I, selfishly, wanted to hear. I wanted to believe that despite obvious physical limitations, life, my life could return to something of normality.

As I awaited my slot in the clinic, I began to feel quite anxious and panicky, and then , this might sound rather dramatic but I can't describe it in any other way, the word "attitude" loomed, in large letters, before my eyes. I could either let this "thing" defeat me, or I could, defeat it! My choice would, certainly , be the latter. I had not worked so hard, in the past years to overcome addiction; to accept how medical misdiagnosis 20 years ago had shaped my life; to meet head on lack of self-confidence and strive for my counselling qualifications AND succeed, despite these recent set-backs. I COULD and WOULD be strong. Life - the quality of my life which I'd fought so hard to attain, would be good again.

I know that dystonia, as my consultant informed me, affects individuals in different ways. Some sufferers only have minor symptoms that interfere very little with their every-day lives and some sufferers receive great relief from their Bot-tox treatment.

There are sufferers out there, such as these two ladies, in great emotional distress and what provision is there for them, other than their three monthly treatments at the Bot-tox clinic? What back up to this is there? I asked was there any counselling support and was told, as yet, not. The consultant did say possibly, a specialist nurse might be trained to administer the injections and give advice on this condition. But will this surely, not be medical advice? Will there be time, in a busy NHS clinic, to sit and listen to ladies, such as these, and find out how they are coping, day to day, on an emotional level.

One of the dystonia sufferers I did contact - his name having been given to me direct from the Dystonia Association Welfare Officer, is a young man in his late 20's. He also had been stigmatised with a psychiatric diagnosis, years before and had, in desperation – his condition deteriorating - made an attempt on his life. Only in the last six months has his condition been correctly diagnosed by a neurologist. I find it incredible, that even now, the medical profession often fail to recognise this condition. When will clinicians see past the labels they impose on an individual and see that this is a "whole person"?

I thank God for those counsellors both in the Addiction Clinic and my own lovely Kate, who did not see me as a symptom but as a whole, living, thinking, feeling person. They, enabled me through self understanding to find dignity, self acceptance, and belief, again, in humanity. They even helped me to learn to love myself, faults and all. If you can't love, forgive or be at peace with yourself, how can you ever give out that love to others? Giving love to others has been the greatest gift, I feel my journey in facing addiction; working towards becoming a counsellor and also, in some inexplicable way, acquiring dystonia, has given me.

Chapter 11.

I return to those tears now, at the beginning of these ramblings and wonder what they were about.

I am no longer sitting, in the warm Italian sunshine overlooking the Amalfi coast line but in my breakfast room at home, looking out on a typical rainy British summer day. Yet somehow, I feel an amazing peace – a peace I find, when I allow myself time "just to be".

Over the past days, of penning this, I have found peace again yet I have also found strength – strength to face the future head on and hopefully, accept, whatever it may bring.

I pray, that you, whatever your situation, may also be able to do this. I pray that if you have a God – be you a Christian, of Jewish Descent; a Buddhist or Sikh, that your God gives you peace and acceptance of any illness, whether acute or chronic, or any other, seemingly, negative situation that has brought chaos into your life or the life of your family.

I am lucky, that my God has enabled and is still enabling me, during the bad days to find that joy and energy for life, that even perhaps, the most able-bodied individual, may not possess. I know that God has been alongside me (though often I couldn't see him) in my journey from childhood into the present and that, although I often can't understand why I seem to be "victim", one day I will see the whole picture and my understanding will be complete.

God (the three in one) has been there for me, in the physical form of, perhaps, the counsellors who opened my eyes and unblocked my ears and when I, in anger, fear or frustration, couldn't respond to human interaction, God lifted me high on his shoulders and kept me safe.

God has been with me throughout this whole and often difficult journey and he's preparing me (even as I sit here) – a stronger, more compassionate person because of personal experience – for the path I should now tread. I trust in Him for my direction.

This has been the story of my psychological and, more especially, spiritual "healing". Perhaps the physical healing will be there for me also some day, but somehow the emphasis – the strong and desperate need I had for this, is now far less.

What's replaced this has been peace and acceptance – acceptance of my illness and a realisation that I can, and will cope whatever my circumstances may be, or become, because God is my rock – the one constant in a continually changing and fluctuating world.

Full Circle.

Part 2: Loss and Retrieval

Chapter 1

It's been a year now, since I've put pen to paper –
busyness, personal difficulties, both
health, family, and   work have left me with both
little time and energy.
It's been a year-long ride on life's roller coaster.
Peaks of pure happiness and
troughs of depression. Depression, not as in the
past – all consuming, invading me to
the core. Maybe, more of a state of unhappiness,
which has been with me a number
of days, ands then I've slowly lifted myself up and
out, of that dark cloud into
something more peaceable and acceptance of life
as it is now.

I'm now on a beautiful Greek island, basking in the
sun
and overlooking the crystal-blue Aegean Sea. Will
this contemplation, space and time
to look back at the past 12 months in clearer
perspective continue? I've now got that

space, which feels so good, which I feel has been lacking in my life in the U.K
.

Perhaps, life,or the pace at which I've been living it, is teaching me a valuable
lesson, once again. I could make this space at home. Yet, perhaps in these past 12
months I've not allowed myself to access this. Perhaps, if I had, the "roller coaster"
ride would not have felt so uncomfortable and out of my control at times.

What I value, so much, about my "new head" since beginning training,
qualifying as a counsellor, is that I'm never going to be too old to develop as an individual
and learn new life-friendly skills.

Maybe, denying myself time to listen to body and particularly mind and soul, has been detrimental to where I now am in life. I have to accept my physical limitations, in order to keep the inner me healthy. This busyness has probably been to prevent me looking too closely at what the future may hold. This is
something I so often challenge clients with from their perspective. How hypocritical
of me! Being too busy can detract from looking too closely at the here and now.It can push
whatever the personal difficulty may be further down, into that place of potential and

dangerous re-assurgance when we are at our lowest ebb. We are then unable to look at it from a
place of rationalisation and realism.

This, perhaps, has been part of my story this year – part of the "dangerous ride" I've allowed myself to travel on. I did develop and most of the time still do have, an acceptance of the illness that has invaded my body and is turning me into a physically premature senior citizen. Yet, alongside this runs a frustration and sadness of the situation.

Initially, the treatment (Bot-tox injections into my neck muscles) did improve my Dystonia but now, it is no longer effective. My consultant feels I have developed immunity to the drug and that the only way forward from here, is medication and in larger doses. If Bot-tox had been successful, then my hope had been, that the medication could be tailed off. I detest taking these drugs (22 tablets per day) as the side-effects are many and varied – blurred vision, affecting both near and long sight; confused thinking; lack of concentration. They all work on the central nervous system, in a slightly different aspect, but the cumulative effect is that each of these side-effects are magnified, the more medication I take. It also takes me back to the toxic medication I took in my teenage years that affected me to the core of my being and changed my personality and identity to extreme.

The dystonia is advancing and mobility is becoming increasingly difficult especially walking. When I walk my involuntary neck movement becomes exaggerated. I have to physically pull my chin down to stop my head turning upwards and to the left to control the spasm. I stumble. I trip. Often my legs begin to falter and join in this "game" of tremor and un-coordination.

The "roller-coaster" ride on which I've traveled has been exhausting both physically and emotionally. My faith, once so strong, has been challenged to the extreme. Somewhere within my subconscious, I know God must be sustaining me for me to be able to carry on, in my role of counsellor. For almost the first time in my life, I believe that I truly do have a talent – a God given talent - that I did not possess before this illness. I believe I am a good counsellor. I can see positive change in clients I have worked with and very often, their feed-back to me, as we close our work, is very affirming.

Please don't think I'm becoming conceited or too self-assured. It this were to happen, I feel the equality of relationship between myself and client would suffer and the process of client empowerment would not come about. I feel privileged to work with my clients and be a party to their often secret and hidden anxieties or concerns. But, sometimes too, I need a "pat on the back" for the energy and emotion I put into these sessions.

Chapter 2

This "second penning" may sound, at this point, a little different from my original script. Is the emphasis more on the negative than the positive? There have been many positive aspects too, over the 12 months, as I look in retrospect. Something that gives me comfort, and this may sound incomprehensible to the reader, is that I do have some control over my ultimate destiny. When I do feel down, when my body feels racked with physical pain and often with this comes emotional pain, I know that there is an ultimate and final solution. Although this is totally introspective and selfish, I have choices still within my life. I can either choose to continue living with a life of progressive disability and its daily consequences, or I can choose, when all energy, (both physical and psychological) is spent, to remove myself, permanently from this, by my own hand. The ultimate choice, I can make, is whether I live or die.

This may not sound a positive aspect, but in some bizarre way, it brings great comfort. It would not be a spur of the moment decision, but one taken with as much consideration to those close to me as possible. Beth would need to be physically and emotionally more mature; education completed and hopefully, in a stable loving and supportive relationship. That is, my role of mother, would have come to a natural conclusion. I also could not commit myself to this voluntary euthanasia whilst my own mother was still alive. The feelings of losing a child, before your own demise, I know can be devastating and I would not subject her to this.

The only questionable factor in this equation is Rob, who is, as described before, badly affected with a hearing impairment. How would he feel, losing his life partner – someone because of his difficulties, he depends on? This is a question to which I cannot find an answer, to justify my potential or future action. I am looking far into the future in this entire scenario. Maybe, I won't reach this point of feeling life has no quality for me. At this point, I can cope with my disability (how I hate that word) despite its limitation and closure on the many physical aspects of life I once so loved. Maybe, the older I grow and see others of my peer group facing similar limitations, the pain will be less intense and more bearable. At this point, I don't know.

Maybe, this time will never come and my life will come to a natural God given closure, without it being by my own hand. Maybe I'll live to be an eccentric octogenarian and even enjoy these late years of my life. Who knows? Only, perhaps God?

I hope the reader can understand the curious, macabre comfort this brings to me, in the here and now. I suppose, if I try to rationalize this, it is to do with me being in control, so different to the earlier years of my life. Control, and choice – these are the aspects that enrich my life and ultimate future, now.

So many events, in the past 12 months, have enriched my life – again in connection with those two powerful descriptive words and to these I would like to add "challenge". Meeting challenges head-on, in the way I never would have previously, has carried me through the difficulties of disability. In fact, the word "challenge" has replaced the word "difficulty" in my internal dictionary.

Challenge has made my life exciting and rewarding and continues to give me energy and drive. Whenever I meet a potential "negative", I try (and most times I succeed) to replace it with something positive, usually a self-set challenge.

Challenge has helped me loose a fear of meeting and communicating with new people. The first great challenge, in to this respect, gave me the confidence to be a speaker at a large gathering of Dystonia sufferers at a conference at Preston, where people came from as far as Scotland to attend. I spoke about how I believe counselling can help sufferers living with chronic illness to regain quality of life. I also led a workshop and a question and answer session.

For some people, this might not sound much of an achievement, but for me, it was something I'd never dreamt of being able to do – the woman who spent a week in her room, during addiction treatment, before feeling safe enough to join in group therapy.

Since the conference, I have spoken to copious Dystonia groups, on the same theme and actually enjoyed the experience. My fear of public speaking has left me. I faced the fear of the original challenge head-on and each successive time, felt my confidence and self-esteem rise to levels I had never imagined possible.

I had returned to horse-riding, as previously described, but began to find it increasingly physically difficult – mostly in connection with my loss of balance. Again, I turned this negative into an extreme positive by joining RDA (Riding for the Disabled) and am taught by instructors who have an understanding of my physical limitations.

I have competed in many dressage competitions in the past six months and actually qualified to compete at the RDA finals in Gloucestershire. This was an incredible experience and made me feel very humble at the difficulties so many disabled riders face, in their lives – blind riders; wheel chair bound riders; individuals with Cystic Fibrosis; riders with limbs missing – the list continues. The atmosphere at the event was amazing – a happiness, excitement, a sense of personal achievement these riders possessed. For me, a wonderful and inspiring scenario.

For so long, I have hated to think of myself a disabled (my mother, sister and family will not use this terminology) but that day, in some strange way, it was a label that I almost felt proud to wear. Here were people achieving and finding real quality of life, despite their circumstances.

I was not even "placed" in my class, but this didn't matter. I did my best and know next year (hopefully qualifying) I'll be back and my riding technique –   different now to riding as an able-bodied competitor – will have improved.

My local RDA is in Clwyd (North Wales), about 30 miles from my home. It is a long way to travel for ¾ hour of instruction, but I receive more from this than just the latter. RDA day (Wednesday) is sacrosanct – no counselling, no catching up with jobs at home. I drive a very short distance to a local railway station and catch an early train to Chester. Armed to the gunnels with riding equipment – hat, stick, waterproofs, packed lunch etc. I make my way slowly (and sometimes painfully) to the bus station where a bus takes me almost to the door of the RDA centre. I have an hour and half to "waste" between train and bus, but even this is enjoyable. Days of rushing from A to B are behind me now, as I wend my careful and slow way through people rushing to their 9 to 5 places of employment. I must look quite

incongruous in jodhpurs and boots amongst all these smart office workers and shop assistants – especially with my head held
at a strange angle and with my weaving gait (walking in a straight line eludes me now!.) Yet embarrassment is not very often in my vocabulary, or has been, in recent months.

If people choose to believe I've consumed copious amounts of early morning alcohol or if they imagine my outward disability is indicative of mental impairment, then, at the point I've now reached, that's O.K.. The only aspect of this, that irritates me (and it has happened on several occasions) is if I inadvertently knock into someone and I get some sarcastic retort, such as, "Can't you look where you're going!" This is actually the problem! Forcing my chin into a forward position enables me to see where my feet are going, so that I don't trip or stumble on pavements or the uneven cobbles. Half an eye (is there such as this!) tries to look ahead to ensure I'm walking in the right direction, but with most of my vision focused downward, this can cause me to bump into people – even lampposts! I often wish I had some equally sarcastic retort to volley back to these impatient individuals, but it's usually well after the event before I think of one.

Nevertheless, I luxuriate in this time between one mode of transport and another and to break up the length of my walk (and here time is on my side), I stop at one of the many early-opening coffee houses in Chester and enjoy a wonderful cappuccino and pastry.

This new, slower pace of life which I originally found quite negative, actually now feels a positive to add to my list. Uninformed individuals may mis-read my outward appearance but, as long as I know the truth, that's all that matters now. And I am convinced that, despite the physical difficulties of my condition, my psychological life-quality is greater than those who make these potentially damaging remarks.

Once I arrive at the pretty Welsh village of Llanfynydd - where my RDA is based, my positive experience continues. The staff who work there (on either a waged or voluntary basis) are very special people. They don't pity or "nanny" the riders because of their disabilities – which can be either learning or physical. Rather, they encourage you to achieve your best, whatever that may be for the individual rider.

The first lessons are mainly for young people with learning impairments – often combined with physical problems also some cannot communicate verbally, in any coherent manner. Yet to see the joy on their faces, the smiles, hearing the laughter, speak volumes to me about their experience. Often a teenager who may have been unable to communicate from birth, begins to use a few words – perhaps the horse's name or an activity connected to the lesson, as physical aspects also improve. A young girl, unable to sit upright without the support of a wheelchair, can now sit up unaided on the horse beneath her. Yes, there are helpers either side, supporting her feet but she too will probably over months find she needs less and less physical support from others.

Many riders come with parents or carers and to see the happiness on the face of the mums or dads as they see this improvement, again, is wonderful to see as an on-looker. Maybe these are only small improvements in their condition (RDA cannot perform miracles) but to mum or dad, they are a small step towards their child becoming a little more independent and improving quality of life for both parent and child.

Chapter 3.

Again, returning to the hustle and bustle of early morning Chester, these hastled, bustling workers in their busy, busy lives miss out on these almost imperceptible mini-miracles.

How lucky I am to be a party to this. I often spend time talking to the mums, dads or carers – maybe with my counsellors's head on? Yet I do feel "off-duty". To listen to their tales and experiences are remarkable. These are not people moaning and groaning about how unfair life has been to them. They are brave, wonderful people, just wanting the best for their child, as any of us do. Their tireless dedication in this pursuit, quite humbles me and touches and enriches my life also.

Some people (my birth family included) are so afraid at looking either physical or psychological illness in the face. Their fear is so great – fear that it might happen to them? Fear of looking at something not "very nice?" I don't know. Maybe, I was once someone like this – pre counsellor training; pre my own illness. Yet, I do hope not. Embracing it myself, head on – accepting that word "disability" does exist (not just for myself, but for others also) has brought such wealth into my life and it's a message I so want to take to others. Chronic illness, physical or mental impairment does not have to bring fore-closure to life quality or achievement. There are many compensations that far outweigh the maybe initially experienced negatives. But one has to get "out there" to embrace and find the positive in this equation.

RDA holds a very special place in my heart and has been a saving grace giving me hope and purpose when I have had to contend with the many losses in life, post chronic illness. My time there each week is something very special to look forward to - a day when all stresses diminish. A day in which both to give and receive; an avenue hitch I would never have been aware of unless the dystonia had not returned. Truly a positive experience.

One can either sit at home and indulge in self-pity, and rant and rave at the unfairness of life or go out and make that effort to find life – a good quality of life, maybe a little changed or different to the former. Maybe, even a better life than the one pre-trauma or illness, because sometimes one's appreciation of what is out there or available, is heightened.

In a similar way, my role of counsellor brings great quality into my life .This is work which I love with a passion and it is difficult to find the right words to express its intimacy and meaning to me.

The initial highlight for me - the end point of three years of difficult academic and practical work - was indeed my Graduation day at Salford

University. I loved it all; my donning of cap and gown; the official photos; the ceremonial "pomp and circumstance" and then the entrance of the dons in their traditional robes. Even the walk onto the stage (head askew) to collect my scroll, in front of friends and family. That was a moment in my life that I never thought I would achieve. A true miracle!

My motivation for entering counselling was to give back what others had given to me. My recovery and re-entry into life began at the A.T.P. Treatment Centre. There, I was listened to; treated as an individual and respected; shown unconditional love (despite some of this being "tough love") and given hope for a better future. In becoming a counsellor, I wanted to be able to help individuals in a similar way, despite their circumstances. Even if others (doctors, CPNs, family) had given up on them, I wanted to help them find something better in their lives, if that was what they wanted. Or, even to gently persuade them that life could be better, if they could not even contemplate this, at that particular testing time.

I am determined I will always counsel whilst I have breath within me and faculties that can be put to gainful use, in the pursuit of giving others the chance of a better life, as was given to me.

After many months of voluntary counselling, I now have a paid position as a Primary Care

Practitioner in North Liverpool. I also work half a day, per week, as a counsellor at a Neurological Centre, helping others with similar conditions as mine. Clients who are coming to terms with recent, often fearful, diagnosees be they acute or chronic Other clients, who may be emotionally "stuck" in the midst of a disease over which they have little or no control. I can relate to both of these scenarios but my time with them is <u>their</u> space and not <u>mine.</u>

Very often, I feel heart-broken when I hear of how individuals and their families cope - or very often don't cope - with life on a day to day basis. Yet, I feel, due to personal experience - both physical and emotional - I have something to give them, even if it only lightens their load ever so slightly. The greatest gift I want to offer them, is that I really want to understand and that I really do care. Sometimes, this gift can merely be space when in a non-judgemental, confidential environment , they can be "real" without putting on a "mask", in order to protect those closest to self.

The personal negative in this, is that, in helping others, my own health has deteriorated quite rapidly. Being a counsellor within the NHS is a stressful occupation. The actual one to one counselling sessions, I find, are immensely rewarding and the very fact, that I am being paid to help others, is an incredible bonus and a great privilege. My overheads as a counsellor are high

- membership of a professional body and needing to undertake professional development courses to maintain this: personal indemnity insurance; supervision fees; the list goes on. I would love to be able to give freely of my time but personal finances do not allow.

Working within the NHS, is not just about reaching out to others in need, it also involves copious amounts of administrative work - monthly statistics to produce; letters to both doctors and clients; long drawn out assessment and discharge reports; personal notes for each client seen etc, etc.

A government agency "Access to Work" (designed to help disabled employees) delivers me directly from home to my place of work, via taxi. They have also provided me with a customised chair which clamps my head in a forward position. Yet, I still get very tired with my case-load and, am in considerable pain at times.

In theory, the counsellor's session with a client is fifty minutes, giving the former ten minutes to complete the appropriate admin. I find this impossible. My medication slows my thought function down and I need time out, between clients, for a break in which I can move around to assist my level of pain. It is also nice to allow time for the occasional visit to the "ladies" or to make a coffee!

The amazing factor in all of this, is that when I am with a client, I become totally energised and absorbed in their situation and can remember scenarios or feelings they have shared with me from sessions, weeks before, which are not even in my personal notes. Yet, when it comes to the administrative side of my work, my brain takes an involuntary "break" and my functioning, in this capacity, is slow and laboured, especially when I am tired.

At present, I am seeing fewer clients than I should - meaning less than an able-bodied counsellor. My greatest fear is that if I am unable to deliver, how safe is my job? .

I won't run, if the going gets difficult, as the "old me" would. I am there to stay. To me, the importance of my role is "to be there" for my clients and put all my efforts into supporting them. This is what my life is about now.

Chapter 4.

I want now to return to the closure of my experience in the Greek Islands. This holiday or 'time out', has been so good. Skiathos is perhaps the most wonderful place I have ever been to - the culture; the people; the natural beauty of the island; the slower pace of life.

I am under no illusion that this is anything more than a holiday and that the return to normality is the testing point. The testing point as to whether the thinking, the feelings I have today, as I sit in the glorious sunshine, listening to the waves gently lapping on the shore – our last few hours in utopia. – will still be intact when I return to my busy life at home.

I'm sure some of these feelings will be diluted, as I experience the drop in temperature, the seemingly endless rain at the tail-end of the British so-called summer. Yet, I also feel, in self-reflection, the essence of my feelings and where, perhaps, my thinking has become sullied in the last few months, will remain with me.

Sometimes I wish I didn't have family who depended on me so much – husband, daughter. This does sound incredibly selfish, but I find that their moods, whether it be anger, frustration - whatever - affect mine also, and I choose to let this cause a dip in my view of the world, in the here and now. Somehow, I have moved on in my life and the way I view it, and they have remained behind. There could be be little truth in my feelings that they want me back to the someone I once was, yet, I still do sometimes sense this. Life, for all of us, would be much less complicated. I don't mean that they want the "addict" back in their lives but, perhaps, they would prefer the person I was prior to my counselling training and personal growth. Life could possibly be, less emotionally arduous for me if I had this facility - this luxury of exclusive time for self and the work in which I am now involved.

I do love them both dearly and especially my thanks go to Robin, who remained alongside me through both the good and the bad times - and believe me the bad times were BAD. The greater and saner part of me says, "I need them as much as they need me. It is my time to support THEM through any future difficulties they now may have."

Rob and I have spent a great part of this holiday looking at the meaning of our relationship and how we both view the world about us. It has brought us closer together in the relaxed atmosphere of the island, but I also feel it has a potential to pull us further apart, when we return to the UK routine. I truly hope not, but it has to do with the aforementioned growth of one partner, leaving the other behind.

I sometimes, feel sad that Rob still can't allow me to have bad days, when I do cry and feel life has dealt me a cruel hand. I need to be honest and feel this experience. I can't and won't "push it down" to make the scenario better for others. My life is based on truth now – a true expression of how I feel and how I think. Sometimes I do need to vocalize this. The difference now, to when I was in psychological turmoil, is that I know that tomorrow is another day and I may wake with entirely different feelings and a sense of real positive anticipation for the future and what it holds for me.

With regard to Beth, I do feel a guilt for her earlier years before I found the "real me". Did I, in the veil of emotional and psychological turmoil, damage her also? I truly hope not. She has grown up into a beautiful, confident young lady, set to go to university and study Law. We do have the usual teenage set-to's , when for an hour or two, she hates me and I can't wait for her to leave home for university.

I often feel, because of the past, I give in too easily to her demands – some kind of emotional payback for the past. Beth knows I'm the "soft touch" compared to her father. Yet in a converse way, there is a ......resentment that life has been so easy, so uncomplicated for her. Beth, sometimes, can't understand the way chronic illness can change lives. But, then again, why should she? The selfish part of me feels a little hurt by this, but the more she matures the more understanding she becomes, but mostly, the altruistic part, feels glad that her life is good and that she lives every enjoyable moment to the full.

I believe I feel this most, because she is at the age when my life and the internal plan I had mapped out for self, crumbled away. I lost my chance to go to university because I was deemed psychologically unfit. I lost my friends and peers because they followed the original plan I would have taken. They became doctors, dentists, vets, teachers, nurses. They found identity in their chosen careers. I became isolated and lost my identity in the various mental institutions to which I was committed.

I took on a new identity – the identity the eminent consultants and psychiatrists labeled me with, that stayed with me until so very recently – a damaging, destructive identity that gave me no hope for the future.

I look at Beth and part of me thanks God that she will get to live out her own internal plans, that will hopefully bring her future happiness. I look at her and I think, "That could have been me", if my condition had been correctly diagnosed in 1972

and seen as a physical (rather than psychological) illness, "I could have had that experience, setting off on a new adventure both of learning and social interaction." How I would have longed for that experience and how I even long for it now. I sound like a selfish, ogre of a parent, resenting my daughter's future. I don't
mean it to come across like this. All I want for Beth, is for her to fulfill her dreams and aspirations, in a way which I couldn't.

Now at the age of 47 years I do have a positive identity and challenges in my life which I want to takle head on. I shouldn't look back and indulge in lost years .I now have a purpose and a future.

Chapter 5.

On this holiday Beth brought two similarly aged female friends with her and they had an amazingly good time I was surprised at myself (and Rob) how liberal we were with them, but then I have to keep reminding myself that they are all nearing the age of adulthood.   Late nights ran into early mornings. The young Greek men were greatly enamored with this bevy of British youth and beauty and were most attentive. Yet to me, the main concern was that they were safe and having fun. Rob I perused the "night scene" in Skiathos town, surreptitiously,   on the first night of our arrival and got a flavour, also, of the male population, be they "native" or tourist. Recounts of their exploits (out of Rob's hearing) were hilarious. One of Beth's friends said she'd never laughed or had such a fun time before.

Fun, laughter, good times are what I feel teenagers should have access to, as long as they do not endanger themselves or others. Sometimes, it feels (and I see this in my counselling work) that no one knows what hardship may be around the corner in life's journey. If joy can be accessed, grab it in both hands, and experience it. This is my new philosophy and I feel it is a healthy one.

I don't want to be a mother who experiences life through her child, but, maybe, there is just a tiny bit of that in me. I suppose I want to know what life can be like for a "normal" 18 year old, because I never experienced that at Beth's age.

It also reminds me of a 17 year old blind rider, whom I met on an RDA holiday this year. Naomi asked me so many questions about Beth, when she knew I had a similarly aged daughter – what she wore; what her 6th form college was like; what she did socially. This made me feel extremely sad and humble. It takes me away from any self-pity in connection with my own lost youth. This teenager was living and experiencing her life in the here and now, not as a memory as in my scenario. Her pain was raw and palpable in its presence. I have chances for a better life ahead of me, even though I am 47 years old. What chance does Naomi have?

Beth and her traveling companions befriended two British boys on the latter days of
the holiday. The day we began our departure for home, I sat with them in their group and chatted with the young people for half an hour or so. One of the boys – a 16 year old – asked if I worked with or spent much time with teenagers because I "spoke" the same language. He was saying this in a complimentary (I asked Beth later!) rather than reproachful manner.

I hadn't realized this before. Is it me reverting to being that young person I was never allowed to be? (The Michael Jackson scenario re:loss of Childhood ? !!) Or is it to do with my recent training, in that I find it easier to "be" with individuals no matter what age, sexual orientation, culture, etc., they may be.

Maybe, it's a mix of the two. Whichever, I feel more confident and more relaxed with individuals and I certainly didn't feel there was anything negative in what this young man said. I took it as a compliment and I'm sure this was how it was intended to be taken.

In the same manner and in relation to my clients, I do find myself adopting their mannerisms, whether in the way in which they sit or in regard to their usage of language. I can be very "prim and proper" with an elderly client, or use language with another that I would never use at home! But this comes somehow in a natural, un-forced way. I don't realize I am doing this, often, until much later, - when, perhaps writing notes in connection to the session. The remark from this young man made me think more about why this happens. I feel it is about meeting the client at the level at which they are, at any certain time and hopefully it fosters a better relationship and one of equality.

As the reader may perceive, training for and qualifying as a counsellor has given me as much as I (hopefully) give to my clients. It is a role I want to be in, for as long as I possibly can help and support the clients I work with. This "learning" has changed me, as an individual, not only in my working life, but also in my family and relationships in the world outside.

Again, I stress it has given me so much – the ability to believe in self; the ability, even to cope with my illness. I just hope and pray daily to God that I can give as much as I have received and continue to receive.

I also know that, even at the age of 47 years, I am still growing, as a whole person, on a daily basis and will continue to do so, until the day I die. THIS I find exciting. Our bodies may grow old and infirm, but our minds, if we so wish, can continue to grow and develop. If this doesn't happen, we have the responsibility and the ability to make it happen.

Further exploration of self, in this manuscript has been a real learning and cathartic experience for me. Committing these thoughts, to paper has hopefully, cleared my mind and made my resolve stronger, to handle whatever the next twelve months (and the future) may bring.

At this point, I feel I want to bring closure to my ramblings. Some of this has been self-indulgent, yet I do hope and pray, within this, that I can bring hope to others in a similar situation.

I stress again, trauma - be it physical or psychological, does not have to bring fore-closure on life quality. But effort, in both these areas does need to be made for positive change to come about. If that effort is not there – life (a life of quality) may not come about, certainly, not by chance, by luck or by destiny. One has to go out into the world and make that supreme effort to find quality and hold fast on to it, whatever is "met" around the next corner.

Believe in yourself and in your potential – even if it is, as yet, un-fulfilled. But above all, dear reader, enjoy your life. We are only in this earthbound place for a short time - make the most of these years Do not die with words of regret on your lips - for experiences not tasted ; for words not spoken.

To return to my title of Part I, "Desperately Seeking Pauline", I might have, at times, lost a little of her essence, in my journey of the past 12 months , but with faith in God and the abilities He has given me ,Pauline (maybe an even stronger one than a year ago and, again, through personal experience) is still there - maturing and growing as an individual. I feel proud to be that person who has found her place and way in life.

Conclusion

It is now nearly three years since I concluded "Full Circle" in its 'e' format and within the last week, my publisher has informed me that it is now going into paperback issue. I wondered whether the reader might like to know the course my life has taken since this time.

I am still employed as a primary care counselor in a large north Liverpool G.P practice and am well settled into this role. My employers have made allowance for my disability and for that I am extremely grateful. I do not work with as many clients per week as my colleagues but feel I put as great an effort as I am able into each working day. I also feel a safety that my employment is as secure as it can be for any of us in this day and age.

It is a challenging occupation but one which I still feel privileged to undertake. I work with a vast range of clients from the anxious single young mum to the 80 year old bereaved grandmother. Each one is special and unique and, hopefully, this is reflected in the way in which we work together.

The ethos of psychological services within the NHS has made a positive change since my experiences of the 1970's. Thankfully, the so called "service user" (that is the patient) is treated with far greater respect and dignity. There is, generally, more parity in the relationship of therapist and client. The latter now has a "voice", is listened to and is, most often, given choices in the direction of treatment. Stigmatization regarding mental health conditions is far less as professionals learn from those they help and even attempt to spread this message to the wider community. On the occasion of my job interview, there was even a service user on the interviewing panel! Has the age of enlightenment finally arrived?

Naturally, nothing is perfect and there will always be flaws in any system, no matter how positive or innovative it may appear. However, in general, I feel proud to play a part in this service and greet this change of direction and thinking with delight.

I derive great satisfaction from working with clients in an attempt to improve their self confidence and esteem. As the reader well knows, this was one of the most difficult issues I, personally, had to tackle over many years. An issue that led me into the dark abyss of depression and, eventually, into addiction.

I feel I am still growing and evolving as an individual and will until I reach my end. My confidence has increased accordingly and I find it difficult to bring to mind the "little mouse" who cowered between bed and radiator, in her hospital room, too terrified to attend group therapy those years before.

During the past number of years, I have held down a responsible job in the community; given lectures on counseling related topics at a range of venues from the Women's Institute to local/regional Dystonia Association venues; even had articles published in both professional journals and popular nationally distributed magazines.

The highlight and greatest challenge for me was when I led a number of workshops onboard a British passenger liner in 2005. Yes, I was terrified as this was a "1st" and I had literally bluffed my way into this opportunity (I have acquired good interview techniques!!) Yet, the fortunately successful experience left me exhilarated and excited, akin to ascending my own highest mountain summit and surviving.

Please don't think that success in life has turned me into a narcissistic egomaniac. My purpose in recounting this is to hopefully convey a message of hope to those who may be struggling at present, that there can be a brighter future ahead no matter what circumstances may be in the here and now.

Years ago, this message would have had little meaning to me, so entrenched was I in my own perceived tragedy. I only hope that I can encourage you with my words. Hence, I reiterate there is a "lot of life out there"- meaningful, pleasurable life – to be experienced but one has to strive to gain positive life quality, sometimes to the

9th degree and beyond.

My physical health is at times an issue and there are days when I do feel down. I am even still prescribed a low maintenance dose of antidepressant. What an admission for a counsellor to make! But I feel that is fine if it enables me to lead a better quality of life long term and I feel no shame in this admission. It even makes me feel more "human" and better qualified to work with my clients. Regarding the healthier ethos of today's mental health services, more individuals suffering from psychological conditions are being employed in different areas of the NHS. I know of one young woman taking medication for bi-polar disorder (the newer terminology for manic depression) who works for the psychological services crisis team. Who better than someone leading a fulfilling, meaningful life with this disorder to help others with perhaps a similar condition? Again, what a message of both acceptance from the establishment and of personal hope for the sufferer.

Personally, I now know that if I do have a bad day and suffer the "poor me" syndrome, it does not necessarily mean that I have to stay in that place. I find this newer thinking encourages me and takes me from there to somewhere better in a shorter space of time. Then I'm up and running again.

This year I reached the grand old age of 50 and

did feel a pang of remorse for being a "late developer" and for years lost. Yet, I know there is nothing I can do to alter the past. I can only look forward to a brighter more challenging future both personally and professionally.

My decision is to live each day to the full and to grow old "disgracefully". I am a lot more out-going now – perhaps the person I was always meant to be. I have pursued those things I was unable to during my teens into early twenties - sung wild, out of tune karaoke songs; jumped off a welsh mountain in tandem paraglide jump; danced into the small hours at discos (or whatever the terminology is nowadays) with peculiar dystonic movements – who cares??);   squeezed myself back into a bikini on holiday; watched the magenta sun both set and rise, within the same 12 hours, on a Mauritian beach; even found myself a (platonic, as far as I was concerned) Rasta toy boy in Barbados much to RT's disdain. Poor RT. I cause him so much embarrassment nowadays with my eccentricity which came with the 50 plus syndrome. Pity about the bank balance also. I have also, as you may have discerned, developed wanderlust and my greatest desire is to explore as much of this great big, exciting world as I can whilst I still have breath in my body and faculties within my brain to appreciate the experience.

My philosophy, now and hopefully to continue, is to make up for time lost and embrace life to its very core. As long as my actions cause no harm to others - even though it might raise a few eyebrows, then surely that's OK. It's taken a long time to think this and even longer to express it but I like being me and I love my life, both the rough and the smooth. The rough times only succeed in perhaps making me a stronger person and in making the smoother times sweeter. I know the "grim reaper" will eventually catch up with me but he'll have to catch me first and what a good time I intend to have in the intervening period!!

So, dear reader, that's me in the year 2006 – an audacious 50 year old with a lot of living to fit into whatever precious years God may further grant me. Each day I count my blessings, for there are many and with this, I dot my last 'i', cross my last 't' and put down my proverbial pen until.........Did I tell you, another ambition of mine is to have a fictional book I have written published........ but that's another story (literally) for another day. Wait and see......You may not have heard the last of me.

Pauline

www.ingramcontent.com/pod-product-compliance
Lightning Source LLC
Chambersburg PA
CBHW022155080426
42734CB00006B/442